praise

Finally, moms have a smart, respected authority figure reassuring us that self-care is not selfish, a pediatrician! Dr. Carissa Stanton shares her personal story of burnout and recovery in Motherhood Makeover so that we can learn from her example. The pressure to self-sacrifice and do too much is strong. I'm grateful for Dr. Stanton's new book to help moms find balance and truly be part of the solution. This book is a support to parents everywhere.

Hunter Clarke-Fields, author of *Raising Good Humans*, creator of Mindful Parenting

The amount of conflicting advice we consume as moms and women is massive. And we are bombarded with the things that we "should" be doing or not be doing. The overwhelm creeps in quickly. Carissa steps in and shares a refreshing perspective that so many of us moms are seeking—a way to trust what our gut is saying deep down. With take home messages that are realistic to put into action, this book will give you a sense of yourself back as both a mom and a human being. Absolutely wonderful.

Lizzie Kieffer, PT, DPT—"Doc Lizzie," Pelvic Physical Therapist and founder of the *Mind Body Core Program*

The highest compliment we can pay a mother is to call her "selfless". Self sacrifice has historically been required to be a "good mom." Not only does this book flip that concept on its head, it gives you the playbook on how to actually do it. A must-read for every mother, parent or caretaker.

Erin Holt—Integrative Nutritionist, CEO and founder of the *Funk'tional Nutritionist*

Dr. Carissa Stanton offers a refreshing and empowering perspective for today's mothers navigating the relentless pressure of comparison, judgment, and information overload. With heartfelt anecdotes and insightful analysis, Dr. Stanton dismantles the myth of perfection, encouraging women to embrace their unique journeys and redefine success on their own terms. This transformative guide not only validates the struggles of motherhood but also inspires readers to find freedom in authenticity, reminding them that there's no one right way to be a mom. Embrace the messy, beautiful reality of motherhood and discover the strength that comes from just being you.

Kerri "Nan" Nachlas, NCS—Certified Pediatric Sleep Consultant and Parent Coach

Carissa offers compassion and empathy in a time when mothers feel immense pressure to do more and to be better. She provides real life, practical examples and tools that feel hopeful and possible, rather than adding to the overwhelm. This book is the exhale that so many mothers are looking for.

Stephanie Risinger, MS, LCMFT—Perinatal Mental Health Therapist, educator, and speaker

motherhood makeover

A Pediatrician's Guide to Reclaiming an Authentic Mothering Journey

Carissa Stanton, MD
with Liz Wolfe, NTP, CPT

MOTHERHOOD MAKEOVER
A Pediatrician's Guide to Reclaiming an Authentic Mothering Journey

Copyright © 2024 by Carissa Stanton, MD

All rights reserved. No part of this book may be reproduced, distributed, or transmitted in any form or by any means, including photocopying, recording, or other electronic or mechanical methods, without the written permission from the publisher or author, except as permitted by U.S. copyright law or in the case of brief quotations embodied in a book review.

Interior Layout and Design by Alice Briggs
Book Cover Design by Abigael Elliott

ISBNs:
979-8-89165-184-5 *Paperback*
979-8-89165-185-2 *Hardback*
979-8-89165-186-9 *E-book*

Published by:
Streamline Books
Kansas City, MO
streamlinebookspublishing.com

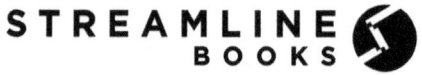

disclaimer

Although the publisher and the author have made every effort to ensure that the information in this book was correct at press time and while this publication is designed to provide accurate information in regard to the subject matter covered, the publisher and the author assume no responsibility for errors, inaccuracies, omissions, or any other inconsistencies herein and hereby disclaim any liability to any party for any loss, damage, or disruption caused by errors or omissions, whether such errors or omissions result from negligence, accident, or any other cause.

The contents of this guide are for informational purposes only and are not a substitute for professional medical advice, diagnosis, or treatment. The author offers no medical diagnoses and/or treatments. Seek the advice of your physician or healthcare professional for treatment of any underlying medical condition before undertaking any diet, supplement, exercise, or other health program. The products and advice in this guide are not intended to diagnose, treat, cure, or prevent any disease and have not been evaluated by the Food and Drug Administration. The author/owner claims no responsibility to any person or entity for any liability, loss, or damage caused or alleged to be caused directly or indirectly as a result of the use, application, or interpretation of the information presented herein.

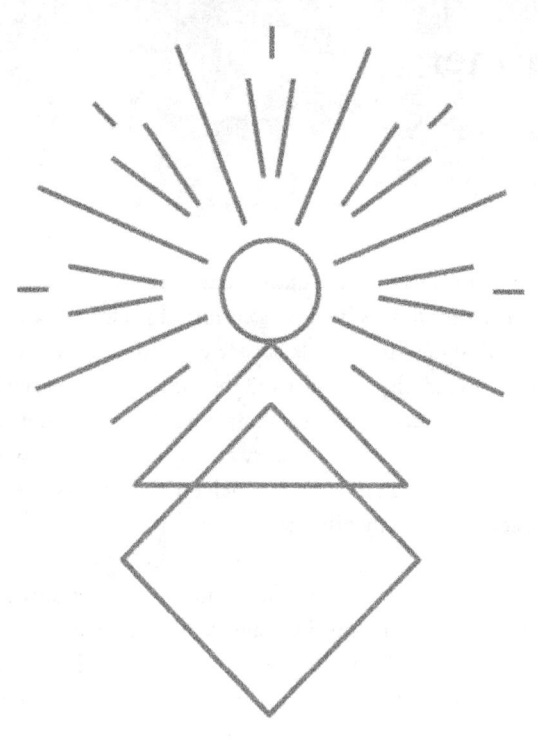

dedication

To all the women caring for others to make the world a better place: may you also care for yourself.

Contents

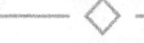

foreword | xi
author's note | xiii
introduction | xv

part I overcome forces working against you | 1

1. you're not the problem; you're the solution | 3
   the problem | 3
   why our cups are empty | 6
   the solution | 8
2. the self-sacrifice narrative | 13
   the illusion of self-sacrifice | 13
   the mirror effect | 14
   the emotional tone of the family | 17
   make space to fill your cup | 18
   we are not robots | 20
3. the more is better narrative | 25
   all aboard the extra train | 25
   human beings not human doings | 27
   create your own culture | 30
4. the unrealistic expectations narrative | 33
   external expectations | 33
   the world does not revolve around the child | 35
   the goal is not happiness | 38
   nurture instead of raise | 40

part II unleash your inner power | 45

5. shed the weight of mom guilt | 47
   the root of mom guilt | 47
   better is okay | 49

fear of missing out (fomo) parenting | 52
secure and sure (sas) parenting | 53
6   weeding through the information overload | 59
discernment | 59
the forest through the trees | 60
fear is counterproductive | 62
control the helicopter | 63
how to weed | 64
7   thrive—not just survive | 69
live to fight another day | 69
stress is not what happens to us | 71
triggered parenting | 73
how to thrive | 76

part III **breakthrough | 81**

8   discover your intuition | 83
mother's sixth sense | 83
find your path to authenticity | 85
parenting is a multiple-choice exam | 87
9   build your village | 91
where has our village gone? | 91
girl talk is important | 93
we aren't meant to do it all | 94
the right village | 96
10 improve your well-being | 99
self-love | 99
cultivate equilibrium | 101
tools for the trenches | 102
11 makeover your motherhood | 113
small shifts make a big difference | 113
you've got this! | 115

acknowledgements | 121

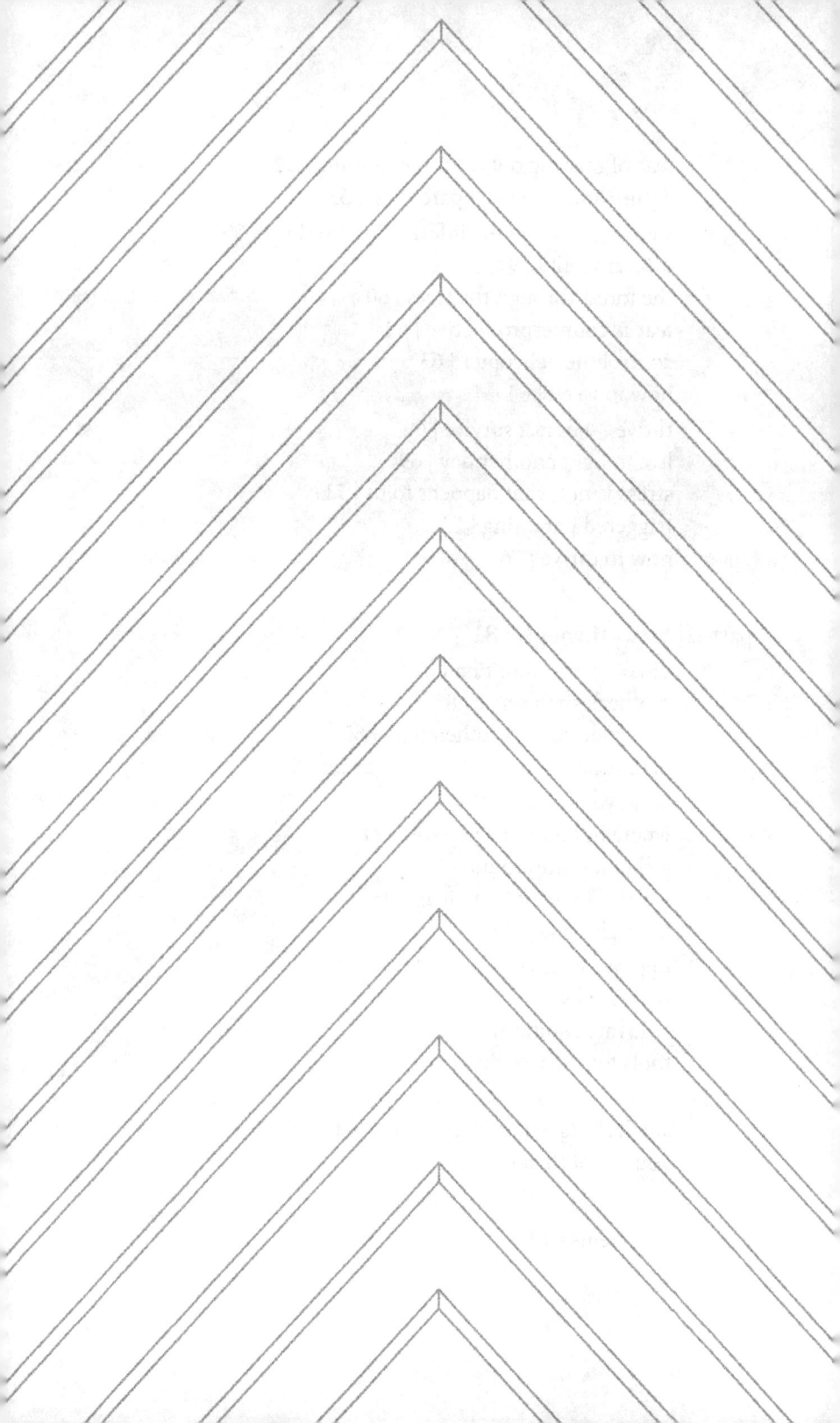

foreword

HEY, MAMA!

If you hesitated to pick up this book, thinking, *Do I really need another "how to parent" book?* I get it.

If you're like me, you've probably got countless "parenting" books on your shelf and in your Kindle. Some you've read, some you haven't; some sit on your shelf *glaring* at you when a situation arises that you *know* could have been avoided had you cracked it open. Am I right?

While I can't *force* you to read this book, I can tell you—this book is different.

It's different because it's not about what you're doing "wrong" or what you could do "better."

It's different because it's not about some "secret" to parenting—whether protocol or philosophy—that only some "expert" knows.

It's different because it isn't about your kids. It's about *you*. (Stick with me...)

When I say this book is about *you,* do you prepare to be judged? To feel deflated or defeated? To be given a long list of "to-dos" to "fix" yourself so you can "fix" your kids?

If so, you need to know that when I say this book is about *you*, what I really mean is that this book is about empowering you to ditch the pervasive, toxic motherhood narrative that permeates all those other books (and courses, and podcasts) so that you can remove the interference, give the heave-ho to the parenting intermediaries and interlopers, and in doing so, swap the lens through which you see the *entire motherhood experience.*

That is what's going to give you back your power and restore your ability to do motherhood with self-trust, inner peace, and alignment with your own intuition.

I speak from experience. That's why I'm here, encouraging you to read this book.

A key player in my own transformation? Dr. Stanton. She's my children's pediatrician, and she's got a heart for mothers as much as she does for children. She has been witness to my process of harnessing my own power, and she's given me the *room* to do so, by insisting—among other things—that *I* am the expert on my own children, and that I have everything I need *already within me* to do this well, with less stress and more joy.

So here's your roadmap for doing just that—reclaiming motherhood, your confidence, your power, and your joy.

Liz Wolfe, NTP, CPT
Certified Nutritional Therapy Practitioner and Personal Trainer
Best-selling author of *Eat the Yolks* and award-winning podcaster of *Balanced Bites*

author's note

AS A MEDICAL provider, I am accustomed to responsibility. But the responsibility of writing a book that anyone can read and interpret with their own lens was a unique challenge. I want to mention some points to keep in mind as you read.

First of all, I've done my best to take into consideration the vast perspectives of mothers and families, but undoubtedly, I have missed a few. Some of the information presented may not apply to you, your children, or your family. One goal of this book is to teach you how to discern if information aligns with you and your family, so it will be a good exercise. Remember there is no right or wrong way, just your way. Use this book like a menu; pick and choose what works for you.

And yes, I am a doctor, but I am not your or your child's doctor. Any advice in this book is general and not specific. Please consult with a medical provider for specific medical advice. At the time of writing this book, I do offer virtual wellness consultations.

There are personal and patient-related stories included for illustrative purposes. All parties have been asked for permission to share their story. Details of the stories may have been changed to keep anonymity, but the general idea is intact.

I want to acknowledge that many of the ideas presented in this book come from the perspective of a developed country that has adequate access to resources. Several of the problems talked about in this book come from a place of privilege, and many people in this world would prefer to have the problems of too many resources instead of too little. The world does have a resource distribution problem. My

motherhood makeover

hope is to help improve the distribution by exposing societal norms that pull modern countries into overconsumption and help people break through those standards.

introduction

"A stirring is happening in mothers all over the world, a desire for a simpler way of living and raising our children. But in reclaiming childhood, we are reclaiming motherhood as well—trusting our instincts and doing what's best for our children rather than what society tells us is normal or expected."

-Ainsley Arment from *A Call of the Wild and Free*

THERE IS A motherhood revolution happening among a generation of mothers who are fighting to reclaim their motherhood experience. I applaud your courage to read this book and join the ranks—I am *with* you, and I wrote this book for *you*.

If we are reclaiming something, that means something was previously lost. Modern society has brought many advantages, but it has also brought difficulties that overshadow and dictate our mothering experience. Outside forces have been allowed to set expectations for us, add more responsibility, and squelch our power. They've taught us to sacrifice our well-being, doubt our confidence, and accept information without question. As a result, modern mothers are feeling disempowered, defeated, overwhelmed, exhausted, unfulfilled, and unwell.

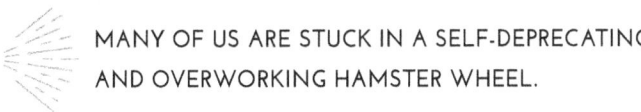

MANY OF US ARE STUCK IN A SELF-DEPRECATING AND OVERWORKING HAMSTER WHEEL.

We cannot continue this downward spiral—there must be a better way. As a result, there is a collective shift in mindset and a rising desire to be more intentional with our own lives, parenting, and family culture. To do this, we will need to resist cultural narratives and discern information to make decisions that align with our values and goals. Most of all, transforming our motherhood experience takes love and care for ourselves to break these cycles.

But if no one has sailed this journey before, how do we know the route to get there? That is what this book will help you find. I hope it will be a way-finder for you, a lighthouse for you to direct your ship towards.

Why is a pediatrician writing a book on motherhood in the first place? I am also a mother. I am in your shoes. With a grown daughter and two stepdaughters, I have overcome many of the same challenges you are facing. I always say my daughters have taught me more than medical school, and it is no exaggeration. Every challenge faced on their journey was a learning opportunity that taught me knowledge and experience to share with other mothers.

Secondly, as a pediatrician, most of my time is spent with the mothers of my patients. Over the course of my twenty-year career, I have spent countless hours listening, empathizing, reassuring, and helping caregivers along their own journey. Along the way they have also taught me wisdom, patience, and understanding. And by observing their trials and tribulations, I have borne witness to the ongoing attack on motherhood. Liz Wolfe is one of those mothers, and I have watched in awe as her courageous journey unfolds—her insights helped bring this book to life.

Last but not least, of course I want to help children. I have learned one of the best ways to do that is by helping their mothers. Let me explain the professional and personal experiences that prompted this revelation. As a pediatrician, I have witnessed firsthand the worsening mental health and wellness of American mothers and children. I concluded this is not a coincidence; a mother's and her children's well-being are connected. I also have personal experience of how my state of being affected my daughter and family. When I was diagnosed with an autoimmune condition that prompted me to take better care of myself, there was a profound impact on my parenting experience and our family dynamics. These events brought an "aha" moment—if I help mothers care for themselves, then I help everyone.

I just need to convince mothers that taking care of themselves is taking care of their children, plus help them navigate the systematic barriers and logistics of making that happen. Talk about dreaming big, right? I decided to start providing wellness consultation services to parents. When I coach parents to take care of themselves, I witness positive changes in not only the parents but also the children. The improvements are powerful and rewarding. Of course I want to spread the word and write a book, so here we are! My hope is I can help break cycles and have an even larger impact—not just for you, but for future generations to come.

For all these reasons, I want to help you by shedding light on the challenges of modern mothering and by giving you insights to improve your experience of motherhood. We have the *power* to make ourselves happier and healthier by realizing that the unreasonable expectations society places on our shoulders are completely—excuse the doctor analogy—treatable.

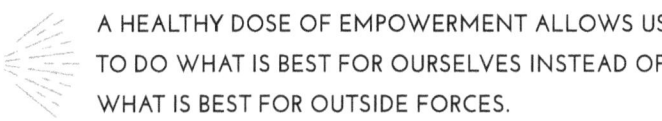

A HEALTHY DOSE OF EMPOWERMENT ALLOWS US TO DO WHAT IS BEST FOR OURSELVES INSTEAD OF WHAT IS BEST FOR OUTSIDE FORCES.

My goal is that this book is something better than a manual and far more helpful than a how-to. When I started researching information for this project, I found insightful parenting books and empowering self-help books. But something was missing—mothers need guidance on how to care for themselves *while* parenting their children in healthy ways.

I am not here to tell you what is right or wrong, but to guide you to find your own way. I approached writing this as if I were talking to you as a client. I will walk you through a self-discovery to connect where you are now with where you want to be. To do this we will help you find the reasons you are stuck, get through those roadblocks, identify your true values and desires, and take steps to reclaim yourself and your motherhood.

The path to get to the destination of a peaceful and sustainable motherhood is different for everyone. Some may undergo a softening and return to traditions and inner self, while others may undertake to strengthen and step into their power. Most likely, the transformation will require a combination of both.

We will embark on this transformative journey in three parts, each focusing on different aspects of your motherhood experience.

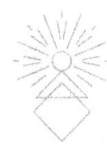

Part I is all about recognizing the forces that are working against you to realize that you're not the problem— you're the solution. Motherhood can be challenging but should not be all consuming; it should not sacrifice our wellness. We'll explore the reasons why mothers' cups are empty, including external barriers that drain our cups. Deeply rooted societal narratives trickle into our daily lives such as self-sacrifice, unrealistic expectations, and more is better, putting the blame on us to feel inadequate, insecure, and burnt out. Overcoming these preconceived notions is key to reclaiming our authentic mothering journey. After all, you are in control and can choose to rise above the outside noise.

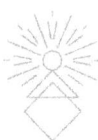

Part II delves into finding your confidence to unleash your inner power. We'll tackle the internal barriers that hold us back, such as information overwhelm, dysregulation, and the dreaded mom guilt. Through practical strategies and insights, we'll help you cultivate self-confidence, trust your instincts, and embrace your unique journey. Building this internal security and assuredness will enable you to navigate the complexities of motherhood with grace and resilience.

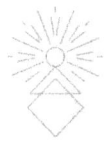
Finally, in **Part III**, we'll put it all together. By breaking through external and internal barriers, you can take steps to makeover your motherhood. I will guide you in integrating the lessons from the previous parts into your everyday life, including how to discover your intuition and build your supportive village. Tips for the trenches is an important section where I share my expertise to improve your wellness. From tools to improve mind-body connection to nutritional insights, I want to give you the information you need to make yourself whole and well.

Throughout the book there will be quotes, personal stories, professional knowledge, and logistics to apply to everyday life. At the end of each chapter is a "Take-Home" section with key points and action items that you can, well, take to your own home. After all, words are just words without enabling action and implementing change.

So, buckle up, mamas! Together, we'll explore the external barriers, cultivate inner confidence, and integrate everything we've learned to make our own version of motherhood. You've got this!

PART I
overcome forces working against you

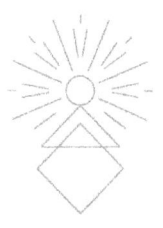

"Motherhood: nothing is quite as hard as helping a person develop his own individuality, especially while you struggle to keep your own."

-Marguerite Kelly

mOTHERHOOD. IT'S A transformative journey that brings immeasurable love and fulfillment. But let's be honest, motherhood can also be immensely challenging, effortful, frustrating, and tiring. It can be validating to admit it is both joyful and painful at the same time—as my spiritual coach wisely reminds me, it's possible to have multiple feelings at once.

The bond between a mother and her child is unlike any other, and it shapes the lives of both in profound ways. And notice I said *both* lives. Everyone focuses on the child's birth and development, and as a society we tend to put the mother on the back burner. But she is going through her own remarkable transformation that is equally, if not more, crucial. Matrescence is the physical, emotional, hormonal, and social transition to becoming a mother—not just during the birth and postpartum periods, but continuing throughout the rest of her life. It's as if we are in a cocoon undergoing constant metamorphosis, literally turning our insides out to rebuild an improved version of ourselves. But the beautiful butterfly that emerges is worth it.

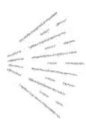

FROM THE MOMENT SHE BRINGS LIFE INTO THIS WORLD, THAT WOMAN WILL NEVER BE THE SAME. SHE WILL MATURE THROUGH EXPERIENCE, GROWTH, AND PERSONAL DEVELOPMENT.

But in contemporary culture, this important process tends to be overshadowed by forces that pressure mothers to sacrifice their well-being, chase unrealistic expectations, and work themselves into exhaustion. Women are finding themselves stalled, frustrated, and unwhole.

It is time to reclaim what has been lost in the modern noise—our unique motherhood experience. The first step is to recognize the external forces that are working against us to make parenting more demanding and holding us back from being our best selves. Then, instead of following a preconceived narrative, we can choose to overcome and rise above it.

CHAPTER 1

you're not the problem; you're the solution

"We cannot solve our problems with the same thinking we used when we created them."

-Albert Einstein

the problem

I have had the privilege of serving as a pediatrician for the past two decades, offering support to countless mothers on their unique journeys. Throughout these years, I have witnessed a distressing trend—the steady decline in the well-being of mothers. I used to see a light in mothers' eyes that is now dimming. Today, when I ask mothers how they're doing, I get a deep sigh, blank stare, or disgruntled response.

Thus I was not surprised, yet still saddened, when I received an alert from the state health department declaring a state of emergency regarding maternal mental illness. The statistics are staggering,

motherhood makeover

heart-wrenching, and illuminating. One in five American women who are pregnant or postpartum will experience a mental health disorder such as depression or anxiety.[1] Shockingly, mental health issues have become the leading cause of maternal mortality, responsible for 23 percent of childbirth-related deaths (in comparison, excessive bleeding accounts for 14 percent of these deaths).[2] Regrettably, if you are a mother in the United States today, you are probably grappling with mental health challenges.

And it's not just mental health, but physical health that is suffering. According to a 2022 survey, 42 percent of women in the United States reported having a chronic disease or condition.[3] Women of reproductive age in the U.S. have some of the highest rates of multiple chronic conditions. Additionally, 80 percent of those with an autoimmune disorder are women, and it is no wonder since an uncontrolled stress response is a known risk factor for these conditions.[4] The mental overwhelm is even overwhelming our bodies.

I know, because I was one of them. I have always encouraged moms to "fill their cups because you can't pour from an empty cup." Yet I must confess that I failed to follow my own advice until I reached a point of burnout and physical distress. At that lowest point, I felt like

---

1 Diana Clarke et al., "Perinatal Mental and Substance Use Disorder" (white paper, Washington, DC: American Psychiatric Association, 2023). https://www.psychiatry.org/getmedia/344c26e2-cdf5-47df-a5d7-a2d444fc1923/APA-CDC-Perinatal-Mental-and-Substance-Use-Disorders-Whitepaper.pdf.
2 Susanna Trost et al., "Pregnancy-Related Deaths: Data from Maternal Mortality Review Committees in 36 US States, 2017-2019." Centers for Disease Control and Prevention, US Department of Health and Human Services, 2022, https://www.cdc.gov/maternal-mortality/media/pdfs/Pregnancy-Related-Deaths-Data-MMRCs-2017-2019-H_1.pdf.
3 Munira Z. Gunja et al., "Health and Health Care for Women of Reproductive Age." Issue Brief, Commonwealth Fund, April 5, 2022, https://www.commonwealthfund.org/publications/issue-briefs/2022/apr/health-and-health-care-women-reproductive-age.
4 Fariha Angum et al., "The Prevalence of Autoimmune Disorders in Women: A Narrative Review." *Cureus.* vol.12, no. 5, 2020.

you're not the problem; you're the solution

a zombie just going through the motions and getting through the day—I was tired of being tired. And my body was too, as evidenced by the disease I developed. After all, if we don't choose to slow down, our body will make the decision for us. In hindsight, I am grateful my body sent me that message. I decided to listen and take action to start prioritizing myself. And when I did start filling my cup, I witnessed remarkable transformations within myself and my family. I realized that by taking care of my own needs, I became part of the *solution* rather than the *problem*.

It took firsthand experience for me to truly comprehend this vital truth: our lives and our children's lives are not mutually exclusive. We affect each other in profound ways both positively and negatively. The mother-child connection should coexist together with mutual give and take, much like other relationships. I learned this the hard way, but I want you to discover this revelation without having to endure harm. I will shout it from the rooftops (or settle for writing it in this book):

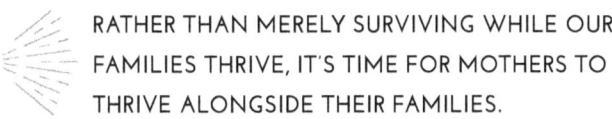
RATHER THAN MERELY SURVIVING WHILE OUR FAMILIES THRIVE, IT'S TIME FOR MOTHERS TO THRIVE ALONGSIDE THEIR FAMILIES.

Motherhood is undeniably one of the most rewarding, yet demanding roles one can undertake. However, challenging does not equal enduring damage. For instance, I often encounter first-time mothers experiencing excruciating pain while breastfeeding. They come into my office with bleeding open sores on their nipples and assume that is a normal part of the process. They confide in me, "I thought it was supposed to be painful," unaware that there is a different, more comfortable experience available to them. I admit I went through this experience with my newborn daughter, despite being a pediatrician in training at the time. I reassure these unsuspecting mothers that while some initial discomfort is normal, breastfeeding should not be intensely painful and cause open sores, and they need to seek help instead of tolerating the pain.

Similarly, in the broader context of motherhood, although having children may not always be comfortable, mothering should not resemble the agony of bleeding nipples. Today, mothers are contending with an unprecedented level of distress—depression, anxiety, loneliness, overwhelm, and burnout have become all too common. This is detrimental to everyone involved and is ultimately unsustainable.

It is evident that something is amiss. Mothers are either burdened with an overwhelming load of responsibilities or lacking the necessary support, and it is likely a combination of both. Change is long overdue. That change begins with you, a mother in the trenches of motherhood, realizing that you are not the problem. Rather, you are the solution. It is time to shift the paradigm and prioritize your *own* well-being *alongside* that of your children.

why our cups are empty

Why has motherhood become such a draining experience for many? It's a question that warrants exploration.

At its core, being a mother is the process of caring for our offspring. It should come somewhat naturally—we are literally wired to do this. During pregnancy and the postpartum period, hormones cause structural and functional changes in our brains and nervous systems to drive us to care for the young by increasing motivation, threat detection, emotions, and social cognition. Evolutionarily, these hormones developed to increase the survival of offspring since the young depend on the mother's efforts. Our brains evolved in ways that increase maternal instincts to empathize with the state of the child—literally wiring a mother's brain to start caring for someone else as much as they do themselves. This is why many pregnant mothers cry at Hallmark commercials, start worrying about random things

you're not the problem; you're the solution

like if a squirrel will attack the baby while on a walk, and start to "nest" their home in anticipation of the baby.

I discovered the power of biology when I was a gestational carrier for my friends. I proudly carried and gave birth to their child. During the pregnancy and birth, even though I knew the child was not mine, I could not help but go through the maternal instincts of preparing to care for a human infant. I even went through the typical "nesting" impulses and made improvements to my home despite knowing the child would not be living there.

This illustrates that becoming a mother can be natural and somewhat *simple* at its core. It is our modern cultural concepts that add extra layers of complexity and challenges. Many of the societal norms of raising children are not rooted in the simple task of caring for them; instead, much of modern parenting has been designed to fulfill society's needs.

Our generation of mothers are facing immense societal pressures that prey on our instinct to care for our children. Subliminal messages bombard us from all directions and brainwash us with their definition of a "good mother." The fast-paced, consumer-driven culture lures us into the trap that more is better for our children. All the while we are sacrificing our own lives to try to keep up with these unattainable standards—frantically making dinner, cleaning the house, buying things to make our family "happy," ensuring our toddler takes a nap, and shuttling everyone to various events. And we're supposed to do it all while enjoying this fleeting moment and maintaining a smile on our face?!

But even with the work and exhaustion, we are inevitably falling short of the illusion of the perfect mother, making us feel inadequate and disheartened. Many mothers are blaming themselves. They're wondering what is "wrong" with them and why they're working so hard without seeing the expected results. What we are experiencing is the definition of frustration: putting in the effort but not having the fulfillment or satisfaction. This is why our cups are empty. And ultimately, it is not our fault.

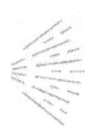

> IT IS CRUCIAL TO ACKNOWLEDGE THAT THE CHALLENGES WE FACE DO NOT SOLELY REFLECT PERSONAL FAILURES OR INADEQUACIES; THEY ARE DEEPLY ROOTED IN SOCIETAL STRUCTURES AND CULTURAL EXPECTATIONS THAT SHAPE OUR EXPERIENCES.

Recognizing the profound impact of societal influences is the first step towards shielding the attack on our instincts and returning to the natural rhythms of motherhood.

the solution

Many mothers find themselves in a place they don't want to be—a disconnection between their current reality and the vision they hold for their motherhood.

The events of 2020 exposed this hardship. During this stressful time many mothers exhibited symptoms of burnout. In the medical profession, burnout is called compassion fatigue or secondary traumatic stress. The condition manifests in mental and physical exhaustion accompanied by negative emotions such as anger, annoyance, intolerance, irritability, bitterness, and resentfulness. Unfortunately, that describes how many of us felt during that time (and possibly still as our society continues to have divisiveness and unrest).

As tumultuous as that time was, it may have had a silver lining. The circumstances forced us to see societal norms we were blindly following, pause to evaluate our situation, and start making changes. We had no choice but to take control and steer the ship in a new direction—it may have been the impetus for change we needed.

you're not the problem; you're the solution

The solution to the problem of mother burnout is *you* and your transformation—a "makeover" that starts from within. Just as a makeover can revitalize our external physical appearance, a motherhood makeover can revitalize us internally to improve our experience as mothers, enabling us to embrace a more authentic version of motherhood. For instance, imagine a woman growing her hair out with the intention of styling it, only to find herself resorting to a messy bun. While the messy bun may serve her fine, it might leave her feeling disappointed and overwhelmed, unable to achieve the desired hairstyle she intended. In this case, the solution may be to opt for a stylish, low-maintenance haircut that fits her lifestyle better.

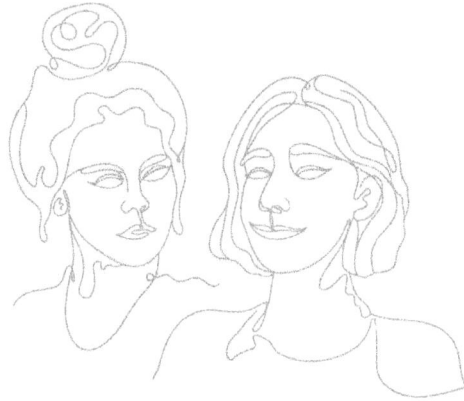

Similarly, in the realm of motherhood, we must identify the areas that are not working for us and find ways to make them work better.

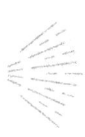
WE NEED TO APPLY A GROWTH MINDSET TO MOTHERING—INSTEAD OF A FIXED MINDSET OF "THIS IS JUST REALITY, AND IT CANNOT BE CHANGED," WE NEED TO REALIZE THAT WE CREATE OUR OWN REALITY AND EXPERIENCE.

Reconciling our ideal version of motherhood necessitates self-reflection, honesty, and the courage to make changes. It's time to peel back the layers that have been added to motherhood and get back to the basics. Just like cutting hair for lower maintenance, you can shape aspects of daily life to fit your motherhood better—and this book will help guide you through the process.

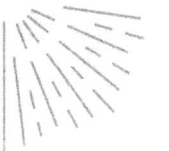 Take Home

CHAPTER 1
you're not the problem; you're the solution

◇ **You are not alone.** Many modern mothers are struggling to have a fulfilling motherhood experience. Being a mother can be difficult, but it should not cause life dysfunction.
- What part of motherhood is the most challenging to you?
- Is that challenge causing dysfunction in your life?

◇ **It is not your fault.** Deeply rooted societal and cultural ideals are working against the natural process of mothering and making it more difficult. It is not that you are inadequate, it is that the expectations and pressures are unattainable.
- What makes you feel most frustrated or inadequate?
- Is that frustration based on the natural process of caring for children?
- If not, what is it based upon?

◇ **You are in control.** You can resist outside noise and pressures to make your own experience. You can decide what and how you would like to parent and make changes accordingly.
- What is your ideal motherhood experience?
- What feelings do you want to have?
- How does that compare with your current experience?

CHAPTER 2
the self-sacrifice narrative

"*What if a responsible mother is not one who shows her children how to slowly die but how to stay wildly alive until the day she dies? What if the call of motherhood is not to be a martyr but to be a model?*"

-Glennon Doyle from book *Untamed*

the illusion of self-sacrifice

Picture this: a tired, worn-out mother stumbles into my office, her energy depleted and her sense of self barely recognizable. Meanwhile, her children seem to have it all—every need and want catered to, as if they were the center of the universe. There's an unmistakable *disconnect* between how mothers care for others versus themselves.

Welcome to the world of modern motherhood, where a prevailing self-sacrifice narrative looms over us. It whispers in our ears that unless we're sacrificing every ounce of ourselves, running on fumes, and feeling perpetually exhausted, we're somehow failing at this whole motherhood gig. Let me tell you, that's a bunch of baloney. Sure, mothers have always made sacrifices for their children. We willingly trade Friday night parties for cozy nights with our little ones. But sacrificing our wellness and wholeness, or losing sight of who we are as individuals? That's where we draw the line.

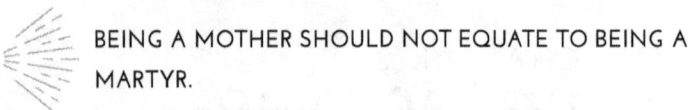
BEING A MOTHER SHOULD NOT EQUATE TO BEING A MARTYR.

Our very self should not be the price to pay for the mere existence of being a mother. Yes, our role as a mother is important—more than a hat you wear or a job you do. But that doesn't mean it has to be all-consuming and dictate your whole life and being.

It's time to break free from the illusion of self-sacrifice and reestablish our own identities without guilt or shame. Mothers deserve to thrive, to care for themselves as much as they care for their children. Let us remember that taking care of ourselves is not a luxury but a necessity. It is not something to be earned or deserved; it is our inherent right as individuals. You are more than just a self-sacrificing figure. You are a person with dreams, desires, and a right to care for yourself.

So, let's debunk the myth that self-sacrifice is the only path to being a good mother. Instead, let's embrace the idea that by nurturing ourselves, we create a foundation of regulation and resilience that can benefit both us and our children. Dear mothers, let's rewrite the narrative. Motherhood does not have to drain our cup; we can make it fill our cup also.

the mirror effect

It is not only mothers who are struggling with their mental health; children are also having difficulties. Recent studies have shown that approximately one in five American children are diagnosed with a mental illness.[5] Recall the statistic I mentioned in the first chapter that one in five American women have a mental health condition. Why are these numbers the same? It is not a coincidence; the answer lies in the mirror effect between mothers and children.

Children learn life skills by watching and imitating their caregivers. They have a remarkable ability to imitate their mothers in various aspects of life. From emotional coping mechanisms and their nervous system state to mannerisms, posture, and habits, children often copy what they observe in their mothers. It's a case of "doing as we do" rather than "doing as we say."

This mirroring behavior is derived from our primitive survival mechanisms. For example, consider the analogy of a mama deer and her fawn feeding in a pasture. When the mother deer is calm and has her head down, peacefully grazing, the baby deer follows suit. However, when the mother deer senses danger, her head and tail perk up, and the baby deer mimics this response. This evolutionary behavior helps the baby deer stay alert to potential threats and survive in its environment.

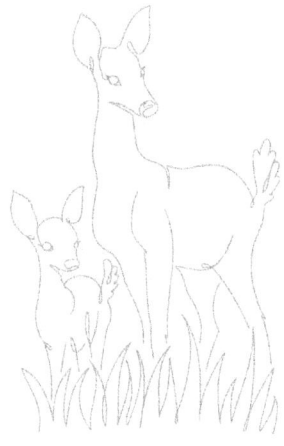

---

5   Rebecca H. Bitsko et al., "Mental Health Surveillance Among Children—United States, 2013–2019," MMWR Supplements vol. 71, no. 2, 2022, 1–42.

Humans have the same instincts programmed deep in our brains and passed evolutionarily. Scientific research has shown evidence of the mirroring effect between mothers and infants. A study focusing on maternal anxiety found that infants tended to cry more when their mothers experienced higher levels of anxiety.[6] It is probable that crying was an outward sign of anxiety they reflected from the mother.

Conversely, there are instances where children have shown improvements when their parents prioritize caring for themselves. Again, we need the mindset that the mother is not the problem but the possible solution.

> One case stands out—a young boy with a facial motor tic that caused him to involuntarily wince when he was emotional or tired. Despite trying various therapies, diets, and supplements, the improvement was limited. However, when the boy's mother sought a wellness consultation and began addressing her own anxiety, a remarkable change occurred. As the mother's nervous system state improved, so did her son's tics. It became evident that the child's condition was closely linked to his mother's well-being. This realization led to a shift in focus from solely treating the child to supporting the mother's wellness. Unfortunately, the previous interventions that were focused on the son, while well-meaning, may have inadvertently exacerbated the situation by causing more stress for the mother. This proves my point: if we help mothers take care of themselves, the positive effects ripple through the entire family.

---

6   Johanna Petzoldt et al., "Maternal Anxiety Disorders Predict Excessive Infant Crying: A Prospective Longitudinal Study," *Archives of Disease in Childhood*, vol. 99, 2014, 800–806.

the self-sacrifice narrative

This understanding of the mirror effect solidifies self-sacrifice as a common yet incorrect belief, otherwise known as a *false* narrative. Unfortunately, past generations of mothers who modeled self-sacrifice passed down a flawed idea. Mothers do not need to make themselves unhappy to make their children happy.

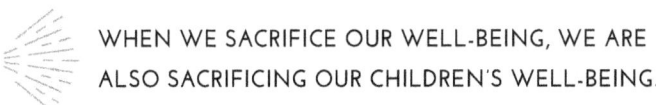 WHEN WE SACRIFICE OUR WELL-BEING, WE ARE ALSO SACRIFICING OUR CHILDREN'S WELL-BEING.

the emotional tone of the family

Think back to a time when your child or partner was struggling in their daily life. How did it affect you? Did you feel at ease or able to enjoy your own day as usual? Probably not. Again, this is instinctual—humans innately want the other people in their group to thrive and are uncomfortable if they are not. It's important to recognize that your family has this instinctual desire for everyone in the family to be well. If one member is not well (including the mother), the other family members have internal uneasiness with this, even if it is not apparent externally. Conversely, if the members of the family are regulated and thriving, then there is resilience in daily life that occurs.

I have personally experienced this. When I was stressed and exhausted, I noticed dissonance in how my family responded to our daily interactions. However, when I made a conscious effort to care for myself and cultivate resilience, we had a more harmonious response to daily life and stressors. The difference was akin to running in tennis shoes instead of high heels—you can do both, but one has more ease to the process.

Mothers, in particular, hold a significant leadership role in setting the emotional tone for the family. Mothers are the wave that initiates the ripple effect throughout the family, shaping the overall emotional atmosphere. It can be a burden at times, but we can also use it to our advantage if we are aware of its power. Therefore it is critical for mothers to prioritize their own fulfillment. When mothers are content, the rest of the family follows suit. The saying "happy wife, happy life" holds some truth in this context.

The irony is that as mothers, we often neglect our own well-being when we are frantically trying to make our children "happy." (In later chapters, I'll explain why happiness may not be the main objective for parenting children.) In the process, we make ourselves less well and whole and contribute to the *opposite* of our intentions. By prioritizing ourselves, we break this cycle and create a more positive environment for our children.

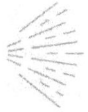 WE CAN PUT AS MUCH EFFORT INTO OUR CHILDREN AS POSSIBLE, BUT IF THE EFFORT IS HINDERING OUR WELLNESS, THEN IT CAN BE COUNTERPRODUCTIVE.

Being an example to our children by demonstrating self-care is the most effective way to teach them to care for themselves. Do we want our daughters to mimic our current habits? Or do we want them to be comfortable setting boundaries, slowing down, and prioritizing their own well-being? By embodying these qualities, we empower our children to live fulfilling lives and nurture themselves.

make space to fill your cup

Motherhood can be a wild and crazy ride, filled with sleepless nights and unpredictable tantrums. Some days the circus music plays loudly in your head as you feel like a ringmaster moving from one circus act to another. It's important to validate ourselves and acknowledge the challenges that come with the territory.

While we can't change the common worries, battles, and ups and downs that come with motherhood, we can focus on what is within our control. We can keep ourselves grounded even if we are pulled

the self-sacrifice narrative

in different directions. It is impossible to eliminate all the stress, but it's possible to make ourselves more resilient.

First and foremost, let's remember that it's not selfish to put ourselves first—it's necessary. Now I know we are not able to do this all the time. If a child comes to us with an injury, we cannot tell them to come back after we do yoga. But we can give ourselves permission to prioritize our needs and recharge our batteries.

I call this "eating the mini cucumbers." Let me explain. You see, I love mini cucumbers, and I buy a bag of them for myself when I go grocery shopping. But often it will be the end of the week and there is my bag of mini cucumbers in the back of the refrigerator, untouched and rotten. I spent all week preparing food for everyone else, and I forgot to cut the cucumbers to eat myself. So don't forget the mini cucumbers for yourself!

One of the most important ways to do this is to make space for yourself. No, I'm not talking about making a "she-shed" with pink curtains and lavender aromatherapy. (Although that sounds lovely and could be part of your makeover plan.)

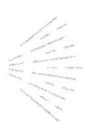
MAKING SPACE FOR YOURSELF IS ABOUT PRIORITIZING RESOURCES (SUCH AS TIME AND ENERGY) USING BOUNDARIES, EXPECTATIONS, SIMPLIFYING, AND DELEGATING.

Think of this process as decluttering your life by changing, decreasing, or removing less necessary aspects, much like you do when you go through your closet to remove unwanted clothes. After all, we are not the Energizer Bunny; we do not keep going and going. We only have so much energy, and for too long mothers have been overextending themselves. It's time to keep some energy for ourselves.

We can start by simplifying and establishing boundaries. When faced with a decision, we can trust our instincts. Is our gut telling us

19

to say no? Would saying yes make us resentful? Saying no to others is like telling yourself "my needs matter." If you are worried about others' reactions, keep in mind it is not our responsibility to make everyone else happy. Those who are truly fit to be in your life will respect your limits—and if they do not then that is their problem, not yours.

This brings me to a confession: I was a people-pleasing addict. I used to dread saying no and worried far too much about what they would think if I did. It was easier for me to say yes, which was a survival mechanism to avoid the fear of disappointing someone. But then I realized not standing up for myself contributed to my unhappiness. When I started setting boundaries and balancing my needs with others, I started to feel more at peace with myself. And as a recovering people-pleasing addict, I can tell you, just like any habit change, it gets easier with time, especially as you feel the positive effects.

The importance of setting limits also applies within our families. It is okay to tell your children no—it does not mean you love them less, but that you also love yourself. The real world won't tell them yes every time, so we need to start utilizing opportunities to set boundaries with our own children. This may apply to a toy they want at the store that will add to our cleaning process or a request for an activity we will need to transport them to. For older children, it may mean telling them they can accomplish a task on their own instead of doing it for them.

Taking care of yourself not only benefits your own well-being but also equips you with the emotional reserves to navigate everyday life. Remember, you can't pour from an empty cup. By investing in your own well-being, you enhance your daily experience. If you're overwhelmed about where to start investing in your wellness, don't worry; I will be giving wellness logistics and tools in chapter 10.

we are not robots

Mothers find themselves in uncharted territory juggling modern responsibilities. One of my clients has a full-time remote job while

the self-sacrifice narrative

caring for an infant and a toddler. I shudder at her stories of timing naps with virtual meetings and waking up hours before sunrise or staying up late to get work done. She is literally doing the work of multiple people.

When mothers are burning the candle at both ends, I give the reminder that we are human; we are not robots. We are not programmed to do it all by ourselves with no needs of our own. Another way to make room for yourself is to decrease the burden we carry by seeking support, delegating, and using shortcuts. Recognizing that we can't do it all and that it's acceptable to ask for help is not a sign of weakness but a recognition of our limitations. (Again, we aren't robots.)

Reaching out to partners, family, friends, or other resources in our community who can lend a helping hand is a step towards creating a more manageable motherhood experience. We can also find "mom hacks" to make tasks and responsibilities more manageable.

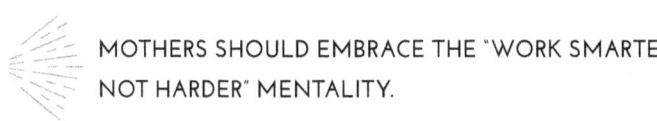

MOTHERS SHOULD EMBRACE THE "WORK SMARTER, NOT HARDER" MENTALITY.

Take inventory of some of your tasks and see if you can find ways to delegate or create shortcuts to make them easier. A common recommendation I give is to find ways to decrease the burden of feeding children, which I am sure you will agree is one of the largest tasks placed on our shoulders. I have seen too many mothers exert unnecessary effort into being a short-order cook and policing the pantry. Pediatrician tip: find ways to simplify and set boundaries with meal and snack time. For instance, I explain to parents the responsibilities of caregivers versus children. Parents should oversee the type of food they provide while the child is in charge of eating the amount of food they want. This simplifies the duty—you just prepare the food, and if your child is hungry, they will eat it. Find what works for you and your family in each season to make mealtime as peaceful as possible.

Now I know what you may be thinking. *If I delegate to others, it may not be done correctly, and then I end up doing double the work.* I hear you. Sometimes it's easier to do it yourself. I have two possible solutions for this concern. First of all, use discernment when delegating—entrusting young children to wash Grandma's heirloom crystal stemware will likely not end well. Secondly, keep in mind, just because the task is not done how you would do it, doesn't mean it's done wrong. If the result is functional then we can accept less than perfect. Letting go of the "perfectionism" expectation is part of the motherhood makeover process.

That brings me to one of my favorite mantras. *"Let it go!"* (as the Disney song says). Let go of the people-pleasing that prevents you from making yourself a priority. Let go of doing everything yourself and not asking for help. In doing so, you'll find that inner peace is attainable, even in the throes of motherhood.

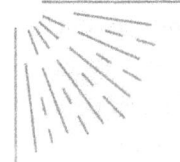

Take Home

CHAPTER 2
the self-sacrifice narrative

◇ **You are not a martyr.** Being a mother does not have to mean sacrificing yourself.
- How were you taught to sacrifice your needs for others' needs?
- How can you change that mindset?

◇ **Taking care of yourself is taking care of your children.** Our children model our behaviors, so if we do not take care of ourselves then they will have negative effects as well.
  - What negative effects have you experienced from lack of self-care?
  - What are the barriers to you taking care of yourself?
  - How can you get through one of those barriers?

◇ **You set the tone for your family.** Our family follows our lead, either positively or negatively. This emphasizes the importance of caring for yourself.
  - Have a meeting with your family and let them know that you will be making some changes to take better care of yourself.
  - Start with a goal to make ten minutes for yourself per day.
  - How does that make you feel?
  - How does your family respond to the changes?

◇ **Make space for yourself.** Declutter your life by setting boundaries, lowering expectations, simplifying, and delegating.
  - Next time you are asked to take on a new responsibility, before reflexively saying yes, reflect if you want to say yes.
  - If you say yes, will that be overextending yourself to meet others' needs?
  - Are you able to say no in this instance; would the consequences be acceptable?
  - Is there a way for you to say yes with stipulations, resulting in compromise?

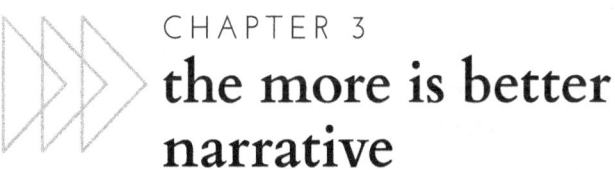

CHAPTER 3
the more is better narrative

"I am a human being, not a human doing."

-Dr. Wayne Dyer

all aboard the extra train

Somewhere along the modern way, mothers have become the all-encompassing "household managers." We find ourselves responsible for juggling schedules, shopping, driving, appointments, homework, forms, and endless other tasks. It's like having dozens of tabs open in our minds, and the mental load can be utterly exhausting. When did mothering become so *extra*?

When I was growing up, I had dance lessons as an extracurricular activity. It was simple and straightforward—class one night a week, an annual competition, and a recital. I remember flipping through a catalog to choose my sequined costume. The experiences taught me lifelong lessons and skills. Thus, when my daughter showed an interest in dance, I was excited to support her. Little did I know what

motherhood makeover

I was signing up for as a dance mom in today's world. Nowadays, dance classes and rehearsals seem to fill up most days of the week. There are multiple competitions and events to attend. The costumes are no longer as simple as picking from a catalog—I found myself spending hours gluing rhinestones onto handmade costumes, one by one. At the time, I didn't question the effort because my daughter was enjoying herself and learning valuable lessons. But looking back I can't help but wonder, did it have to be so extra? Could she have still enjoyed it and learned those lessons without my spending all those hours bedazzling costumes?

Now, don't get me wrong—I'm not saying dance moms are bad parents. In fact the ones I know are mom warriors. I'm not questioning the importance of extracurricular activities, but I am examining whether it should require so much work on the part of parents to achieve the desired effect for our children.

When I talk to other parents about this modern-day "extra" phenomenon, I often mention *Babies,* a documentary from 2010.[7] The film follows four families from different countries—America, Mongolia, Namibia, and Japan. In one scene, the American family takes their toddler to a music class, but the child is not participating and instead walks away from the group to tap her hand on the exit door as if to signal her desire to leave. Then the scene shifts to Africa, where a group of women are singing and clapping in a hut. A toddler walks over and starts clapping and dancing along.

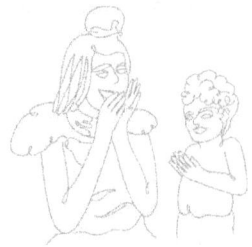

---

7 *Babies,* directed by Thomas Balmès (Focus Features, 2010).

It makes me wonder—how did we go from those impromptu gatherings of singing and dancing, where children could voluntarily join in, to carting our kids around from activity to activity? Was there something wrong with those spontaneous tribal ways? Or is the way we parent today fulfilling someone else's agenda and purpose?

These are the questions that cross my mind as I scrutinize the current dilemma imposed on families.

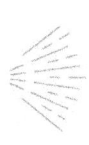

> NOT ONLY ARE CHILDREN OVERSTIMULATED WITH AN OVERABUNDANCE OF POSSESSIONS AND ACTIVITIES, BUT MOTHERS ARE DEPLETED AS THEY EXPEND TIME, MONEY, AND ENERGY TO MAINTAIN THAT LEVEL OF PLENTITUDE.

Society now portrays mothers as messy bun-wearing, exhausted, soccer moms driving frantically in their minivans to the next kids' activity, as if this is the norm we should strive for. My best friend calls this cultural norm the "Extra Train"—we jokingly say, "All aboard! Choo-choo!" when a new duty is added to our ever-growing list.

When we find ourselves on the modern parenting express, how do we slow down and unload? It is an ongoing process to prioritize and set boundaries with our family's obligations. We need to be intentional with commitments and assess if they are truly necessary and beneficial for our family, or if they are taking away from the simple joys and natural experiences that we could have.

human beings not human doings

I often like to say to my young patients, "Tell me about your day." During one particular Monday appointment, a ten-year-old boy told me about his Sunday. His response left me wide-eyed:

"Two baseball games, a soccer game, two friend's birthday parties, and I wrote a book report that was due on Monday." Now, I'm not here to judge his parents; I understand this is our cultural norm. But I was saddened that his description was not age appropriate. He did not describe the events as a child would experience them such as "I played at the park with my friends" or "I read a book about dragons." Instead he rattled off an adult-like series of tasks.

Parenting has turned into this never-ending checklist of activities, where we just go from one box to the next, checking them off.

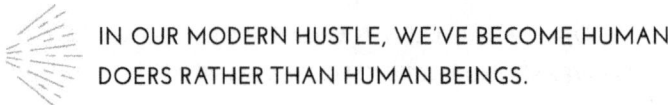

IN OUR MODERN HUSTLE, WE'VE BECOME HUMAN DOERS RATHER THAN HUMAN BEINGS.

We've become preoccupied with our to-do list, causing us to be disconnected from what is important. What we really need is the opposite—to do less and connect more. Then we can have down time for the simple things like lying on the floor with our infant, swinging our toddler around like an airplane, or having tea parties and dinosaur hunts. These things are not only important ways for parents and children to enjoy each other, but are vital for physical, social, and emotional development.

In parts of the developed world, we seem to have adopted a childhood that insists on the never-ending pursuit of more. The prevailing narrative tells us that we must provide our children with an abundance of everything to ensure their success. More activities, more toys, more classes, more assignments, more experiences—there's an unrelenting pressure to overload our children with every opportunity under the sun. The idea behind this compulsion is "more is better," but in reality, too much of a good thing can be detrimental to a child.

Does more truly equate to better? Is there a point where "more" can be counterproductive or even harmful? Just because we can do more, does that mean we should? Here is my professional opinion: more is not necessarily better. In fact, children often do better with less as they feel more secure and stable when they are not overwhelmed

the more is better narrative

with a packed schedule, cluttered home, and lack of freedom. We are not the only ones who need to fill our cup—our children do also.

Kim John Payne explores this concept in his book *Simplicity Parenting*.[8] He writes about how the commercialism and "hyper-capitalism" of our society is pressuring us to rush through crazy daily routines of work and consumption. This, according to Payne, has waged a "war on childhood," where the pace of our lives no longer aligns with the pace of childhood. His solution? To "declutter" childhood. And by decluttering childhood, we also declutter motherhood.

A cluttered childhood can not only put stress on the children; it also puts stress on the family. Mothers have become their children's personal managers—juggling schedules, chauffeuring to activities, making appointments, and tutoring homework, not to mention we still have to parent in between it all. Mothering is hard enough without having to slate it into a schedule. (I'm not kidding, I have had mothers make calendar events such as "teach shoe tying.") This mental and physical overload has caused "modern mom victim mentality" where mothers assume a fixed mindset that this is the torturous hand they've been dealt. I'm here to remind you to shift to a growth mindset—you are in control of your life.

> I was working with a mom who was struggling to persuade her child to practice a musical instrument and attend lessons. When I asked her the reasoning behind the lessons, she said, "Well, he *has* to learn to play a musical instrument to help brain development." Her thought process had some reasonable basis; music can be beneficial for brain development. But I explained it does not have to be in the form of formal lessons, which can be

---

8   Kim John Payne, *Simplicity Parenting: Using the Extraordinary Power of Less to Raise Calmer, Happier, and More Secure Kids* (New York: Ballantine Books, 2010).

counterproductive if the child is not enjoying the activity. Singing around the house, free play on instruments, and even listening to music can be just as beneficial. By simplifying and decluttering, both the mom and the child could find joy in the process.

In the end, we need to remember that it's not about how many activities we can fit into a day or how many boxes we can check off. Just like we are doing with our motherhood, we need to peel back the layers of childhood and get back to the *basics*: creating meaningful connections, allowing our children to explore their interests in a balanced way, and finding joy in the journey of parenting. Our motherhood and their childhood go hand in hand, so to makeover one, we also need to work on the other.

create your own culture

Changing an entire society's culture is undoubtedly challenging and time-consuming. How can we do something different within our families while still living in current society? Start with small shifts at the individual level and be intentional about choices, even if it means swimming against the current.

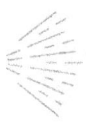

CREATING YOUR OWN CULTURE MAY NOT BE THE PATH OF LEAST RESISTANCE, BUT IT WILL BE THE PATH OF MOST FULFILLMENT, NOT ONLY FOR THIS GENERATION BUT FOR GENERATIONS TO COME.

However, making these shifts doesn't mean you have to uproot your life and move to a remote area or another country, although those options may be tempting at times. You can make small changes right where you are. In her book *Old-Fashioned on Purpose*, Jill Winger writes, "This is a conscious choice we've made to reclaim meaningful ideas that have been discarded in the name of progress and restore them to a place of value in our modern day-to-day."⁹

For example, in my own family, we try to instill certain "old-fashioned" values. We put limits on technology, prioritize making our own food, have downtime in our schedules, tend to a vegetable garden, air dry our clothes, and spend time outdoors. However, our children still have cell phones, drive cars, occasionally get takeout, and participate in typical extracurricular activities. The trick is to find your own balance of both worlds.

I have seen examples in my patients' families as well. One of my families moved from their suburban house to live in a duplex with their grandmother as the neighbor. The grandmother gets the benefit of family involvement, and the family gets the benefit of grandmother's traditions and wisdoms. Another mother chose to decrease the number of scheduled activities for her older children and in place had them take turns making dinner for the family in the evenings. And back to my own example of my daughter's involvement in dance—we chose a team that did not travel and only did the minimum number of activities.

It's important to understand that you don't have to choose one extreme or the other. There is a vast range of possibilities that you can explore and utilize. Our culture often pushes us towards an "all or nothing" mindset, where we feel the need to label ourselves and rely on specific parenting styles or philosophies. I often hear parents say, "Oh, I can't do that because I'm an (insert label) parent." We forget that we can create our own path and be the type of parent we want to be; the only label we need is our own.

In the midst of this modern pressure, keep in mind that quality trumps quantity. Instead of mindlessly piling on activities, we should focus on creating meaningful experiences and fostering genuine connections. It's about finding the level of meeting our children's needs

---

9 Jill Winger, *Old-Fashioned on Purpose* (Toronto: Park Row Books, 2022).

without overwhelming them or ourselves. We should make intentional choices; after all, we dictate our own family's culture.

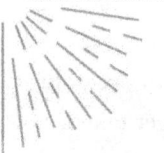

Take Home

CHAPTER 3
the more is better narrative

◇ **Mothering does not need to be all consuming.** You can prioritize and set boundaries.
- **Think about your train "load"—schedules, consumption, tasks.**
- **Brainstorm two ways to lighten the load.**

◇ **More does not necessarily mean better.** Parents and children both struggle when they are overwhelmed and overstimulated.
- **What is a commitment that is decreasing connection with your children?**
- **How can you declutter that commitment to improve connection?**

◇ **You can make changes within your own family to simplify.** Even if society does not change as a whole, you can make your own culture.
- **What are two old fashioned values you would like to instill in your children?**
- **How can you make changes in your daily life using those values?**

CHAPTER 4
the unrealistic expectations narrative

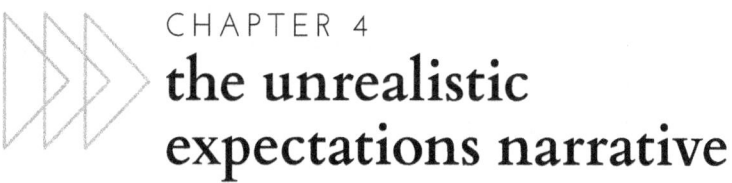

"Disappointment is the gap that exists between expectations and reality."
-John C. Maxwell

external expectations

I will never forget a mother's revelation as we discussed ways to simplify and make space for herself. She said, "I wish I could move my family to a deserted island." What this mother desires to escape are the insurmountable expectations thrown at mothers from all directions. Modern society continues to add more and more burden onto our shoulders while we are being crushed under the load.

I admit, as a pediatrician, I initially fell into this trap. At the beginning of my career, I was taught to throw my "expert" opinion at parents, which is called *anticipatory guidance* in the medical field. For each age group, I had a list of recommendations I told parents was the "right" way to do something. For instance, I used to endorse the standard modern way of starting solid foods in infants—spoon-feeding pureed food. There is nothing necessarily wrong with that, but I later learned there are other acceptable methods. When I started my own practice, I was able to spend more time with mothers and learn their unique experiences and choices. It turns out mothers are already doing their best, and it is rare I need to direct them in a different direction while listening to them. In fact, many times I learn *from* mothers, methods such as baby-led feeding instead of spoon-feeding purees. Ultimately, my checklist was adding more stress to their lives, pushing them away from their own intuition and causing unnecessary anxiety. I was unintentionally perpetuating the same pressures that society imposes on mothers. It was a wake-up call for me to change my approach—it became clear that what feels right for each mother is the "right" way.

Just as I was once telling mothers what they should do, society as a whole tends to dictate what mothering entails, instead of allowing mothers to define it for themselves. Jessica Grose, in her book *Screaming on the Inside: The Unsustainability of American Motherhood*, brilliantly points out how these societal ideals do not serve mothers and their families.[10] She highlights not only how absurd, individualistic, and superficial these pressures can be, but how "they have nothing to do with your private relationship with your own children, your values, or your needs."

Mothers have obediently followed these ideals, falsely believing they are in the best interest of our children. But the impact of following external expectations is starting to come to light. Case in point, a narrative that hovers over parents is to cater to our children's happiness and shield them from any discomfort. In reality, this approach is counterproductive to developing independent, functional, and resilient adults, which is the ultimate goal of parenting. How are we supposed to coddle them and, at the same time, equip them to face

---

10 Jessica Grose, *Screaming on the Inside: The Unsustainability of American Motherhood* (New York: Mariner Books, 2023).

life's adversities? Society is asking mothers to do the *impossible*. No wonder we are tired! Where there are expectations, there is bound to be disappointment.

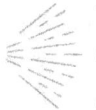 **WE ARE REALIZING SOCIETAL STANDARDS ARE NOT ONLY UNHELPFUL BUT IN FACT HARMFUL TO US AND OUR FAMILIES.**

It's time for a rally cry. We will no longer dutifully follow precedents set for us by others. It is our turn to tell society what *we* want.

the world does not revolve around the child

What do we want? Ultimately, that is up to you. But I believe we all want the same underlying goal; we want to do the best we can for our children. Society, though, has absurd expectations for what parenting "the best we can" entails, putting mothers into tailspin as we scramble to implement these ideals.

Until recently, humans had approached parenting from a family-centered perspective, involving the children in the family unit's best interests. However, modern developments have once again prioritized society's best interests and shifted our focus to child-centered parenting with the misconception that we must do everything for our child. This misguided notion has driven us to the point of exhaustion as we tirelessly strive to meet unrealistic expectations.

One way I try to solve "modern" problems is to look back at the "old days." During my visits to places with more ancestral or native cultures, I've witnessed different approaches to parenting. In most of these instances, the children are more involved in day-to-day life. For instance, in Rwanda I witnessed mothers tending to the crop fields while their children picked up rocks to throw out of the field. The children seemed content with rock-throwing as a form of play, but it also helped to clear the field for planting.

It's disheartening to see how we've lost some valuable ancestral philosophies in modern times. I believe we could benefit from re-adopting some of these pearls of wisdom, and I'm not alone in this sentiment. In Michaeleen Doucleff's book *Hunt, Gather, Parent*, she embarks on a global journey to explore how other cultures approach parenting and why the modern ways are damaging to children and their parents.[11] Through her research, she uncovers significant differences in how children play, learn, do chores, build confidence, and deal with emotions across cultures.

For instance, in native cultures, children are seen as productive contributors to the family's everyday life, such as my story of children throwing rocks from the crop field in Rwanda. This involvement benefits both the children and their parents—the adults are able to complete their daily tasks while the children are fulfilled doing their part. Even America started this way—think of the pioneer children helping with farm chores.

In contrast, contemporary culture has convinced parents that their main responsibility is to shield their children from anything that distracts them from child-focused activities. There is a misunderstanding that children can only learn from activities such as play, schoolwork, and activities that are specifically geared toward them. This expectation exhausts parents who are acting as their child's servants, shouldering all the household chores *and* expending resources (time and money) to entertain their children. Furthermore, the approach is a disservice for our children by undermining opportunities for freedom, personal value, and skill building. Sheltering our kids from tasks and chores is inadvertently creating a generation of children who are less capable of independence.

---

11 Michaeleen Doucleff, *Hunt, Gather, Parent: What Ancient Cultures Can Teach Us About the Lost Art of Raising Happy, Helpful Little Humans* (New York: Avid Reader Press/Simon & Schuster, 2021).

the unrealistic expectations narrative

When my daughter was graduating high school and preparing to leave our home, I realized there were life skills that she had not yet learned such as doing laundry and unclogging a toilet. Teaching her became yet another checklist and additional responsibility for me to complete. In hindsight, we should have been involving her in the day-to-day tasks so she could learn along the way, instead of playing catch up in adolescence.

> On the other hand, when my daughter's friend from Botswana stayed in our home, I witnessed firsthand the difference in cultural upbringing. He was more willing to help and contribute to household functions. When he saw a chore that needed to be done, he would do the task without being asked. This is not a common occurrence in my family (in my family's defense, that is what our culture dictated and how we allowed them to be taught). He explained that during his childhood the family involved him in chores and daily activities starting at an early age and expected him to contribute to the household functions. As a result, he has positive attributes such as confidence, capability, and resiliency that were instilled from his family's way of life.

You've probably heard the older generation say, "When I was a kid, I walked to school in the rain, uphill both ways," pointing out how future generations have it easier. Now it seems that as children have it easier, parents have it harder. Modern mothers are doing more and more for their children, leaving the children less competent and resilient.

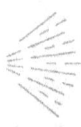

> IT IS TIME TO SHIFT THE FOCUS AND INVOLVE THE CHILDREN IN EVERYDAY LIFE, DOING OUR ACTIVITIES OF DAILY LIVING *WITH* THEM, INSTEAD OF *FOR* THEM.

the goal is not happiness

We don't want our children to be unhappy, or do we? We must question whether the modern goal of children's happiness truly serves the best interest of both parents and children. A fulfilling life is not solely derived from the absence of discomfort. It is through experiencing challenges, making mistakes safely, and having a sense of purpose that our children can truly thrive.

From a pediatric standpoint, it has been proven that developmentally appropriate challenges increase resilience in children.[12] Resilience is the ability to adapt to challenges and is an important skill to acquire to navigate life successfully. In childhood, exposure and overcoming minor stressors can help a child prepare to handle larger stressors later in life. However, our culture discourages discomfort, which infers that difficulties should be avoided. To counteract this notion, I often use the immune system as an analogy. As a child is exposed to common germs, the immune system develops antibodies and becomes more able to fight future germs encountered. If a child is not exposed to germs, then the immune system may not be as ready and equipped to counteract future threats. Just like the immune system, our child's brain needs to be challenged to learn how to handle future challenges.

Overcoming discomfort and difficulties can also be beneficial to a child's esteem by increasing belief in themselves. If someone solved all your problems for you, how would you feel? As glorious as that

---

12 Ann S. Masten and Andrew J. Barnes, "Resilience in Children: Developmental Perspectives," *Children (Basel)* 5, no. 7 (2018): 98.

sounds in the present moment, eventually it would negatively impact your confidence and self-awareness. If you've ever sustained an injury that impeded your function and become frustrated with your inability to do something yourself, you know the feeling children can have when we do everything for them.

When I need to be reminded of this, I think of my grandmother who successfully raised twelve children. She spent most of her days in the kitchen, but whenever a child was hurt or faced a problem, they would enter the kitchen, and she was always there for them with a kiss on a booboo or an empathetic ear. For the most part, that's all they needed. She was calm and secure, knowing these little trials were part of the process of growing up. I often draw upon this memory when I feel overwhelmed. I ask myself if I am being a consultant who allows my children to come to me for help or a hovering helicopter swooping down to the rescue at the sign of any "unhappiness."

Unfortunately, many children are going through an abnormal lack of adversity with modern parenting. We must keep in mind that it is not the discomfort that negatively impacts the child, it is being alone in that discomfort that can. As long as the child has your support, feeling discomfort can actually be *beneficial* to their development and wholeness. When a parent is uncomfortable with their child's discomfort, it is often the parent that needs to address their own discomfort first.

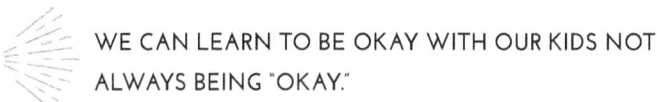

WE CAN LEARN TO BE OKAY WITH OUR KIDS NOT ALWAYS BEING "OKAY."

Scrambling to fulfill our child's every want and whim is like chasing a moving target, which will ultimately lead to disappointment when we fall short. After all, happiness is a feeling, and we are not responsible for other people's feelings. We need to absolve ourselves of the unreasonable duty to make our children happy.

▷ nurture instead of raise

I've never been a fan of the term "raising children"; it implies the parents are doing the work of lifting them up. Instead we are simply providing an environment that allows them to grow and thrive. Much like a gardener does with a plant, we provide the soil, water, and sun; but ultimately, it is the plant that does the work. When it comes to parenting, sometimes being more passive than active can yield remarkable results. Unfortunately, the expectation placed on modern parents is to be overly involved in their child's life.

WE NEED TO FOCUS ON NURTURING OUR CHILDREN BY GIVING THEM THE FREEDOM TO DEVELOP, WHILE ALSO BEING TRUSTED CONSULTANTS WHENEVER THEY NEED GUIDANCE.

I often use a simple analogy to explain this concept to parents. I tell them that their child's journey of growing up is like driving on a road. Along the way, there will be bumps, detours, and unexpected turns, such as learning to walk, starting school, or going through puberty. As parents, we are like the guardrails on the side of the road. It's okay if our child veers a little while they adjust to the new terrain. However, if they start driving off the road completely, we step in to provide guidance and help them find their way back.

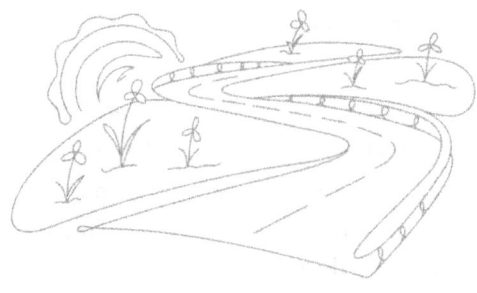

the unrealistic expectations narrative

Just like we can't bulldoze clear the road they travel on, we are not responsible for alleviating the challenges they will encounter. Our role as parents is not to micromanage their every move, but rather to be there as a steady presence, offering support and guidance when needed. It is our duty to make sure our caring does not become coddling.

We can find ways to shift our parenting from raising to nurturing. A story from my daughter's childhood comes to mind to illustrate this point. One morning, in the middle of winter, she decided she wanted to wear a skirt to school. After I explained the cold weather forecast and pointed out she had outdoor recess, she still insisted on wearing the skirt. I took a deep breath and realized she wouldn't be harmed by this decision, so I allowed her to "veer off" her lane and wear the skirt. She not only survived recess; to this day she always checks the weather before getting dressed. By letting go of the unrealistic expectation that I control her happiness and outcomes, I allowed her space to feel discomfort, and she learned on her own.

I know what you are thinking—it is more comfortable to be in control. Many modern parents fear letting go of the steering wheel. There are numerous factors weighing into this, including the pressure on parents and children to live up to unattainable standards. Often what we expect from children is beyond their developmental abilities, causing parents to need to swoop in and assist. If we scale back these expectations to match their maturity level, then the child is able to handle them on their own.

Another factor that comes into play is the cultural idea that adults are in charge of their child's success (or lack thereof), again taking the stance that we are the ones doing the work of "raising" the children. It would be reassuring if this was the case. But again, that control is an illusion, creates more work, and may not be in the best interest of the child.

The opposite end of the spectrum is allowing the child to be in control. Passively parenting by allowing the child to lead gives them responsibility they are not ready to handle, which can cause dysfunctional behavior. Though we cannot control every move a child makes, we can set boundaries to absolve the child of responsibilities. For instance, we cannot force them to fall asleep, but we can set the boundary of having them in their bed at a set time. Once again, we have to find our happy medium.

Letting your child find their path is easier said than done; after all, we love our children more than anything. But what if we realize that the best way to love them is to step back and give them room to grow? Making transitions to this approach will give you and your child more peace and freedom. When I feel myself getting stressed to meet unreachable standards or trying to control my child, I whisper this phrase to myself: "Lower the bar." It's time to lower the bar of expectations placed on mothers.

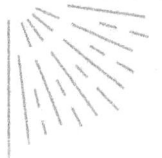

Take Home

CHAPTER 4
the unrealistic expectations narrative

◇ **Social norms do not define you or your family.** You can set your own standards that align with your connection to your children, values, and personal needs.
- List your top priorities and expectations as a mother.
- Now list what external expectations you may be chasing.
- Compare the list and find ways to live up to your list instead of the external list.

◇ **Ancestral parenting revolved around the needs of the family, whereas modern parenting revolves around the needs of the child.** Involving children in daily tasks can be helpful for the parents and the children.
- What daily task can you involve your children with?
- What barriers are there to involving your children instead of doing it for them?
- How can you get through those barriers?

◇ **Focusing your efforts on children's happiness is futile.** Chasing a goal of happiness will exhaust and frustrate parents, and children need to be allowed discomfort and challenges to learn resilience. We need to be comfortable with our children being uncomfortable at times.
- Think of the last time your child was uncomfortable.
- How did you feel?

- What did you do?
- Were you willing and able to allow them the space to work through that discomfort?
- What can you do to allow them more space?

◇ **Despite what our culture perpetuates, parenting should be more passive than active.** We should give our children the tools they need and help guide them along the way, but we are not in control of their everyday lives. Relinquishing responsibility for our child's outcomes will decrease our stress and improve their competency. Remember you can be a guardrail; allow them to find their path but be ready to guide them back on track if needed.

- Next time your child is faced with a challenge, consider whether you can allow them to work through it on their own.
- Do they have the maturity level to handle the situation?
- Is the situation not harmful to themselves or others?
- Would the possible results be tolerable?

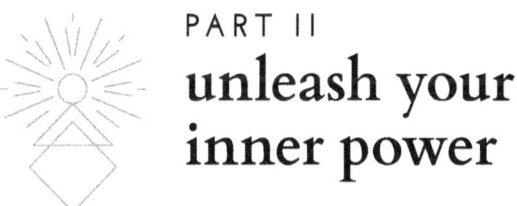

PART II
unleash your inner power

"You've always had the power, my dear, you just had to learn it for yourself."
-Glinda to Dorothy in Wizard of Oz

iN PART II, we will turn inward, uncover what undermines our power, and discover ways to rebuild it. Empowerment is the incredible process of harnessing your inner strength and cultivating unwavering confidence. It's the foundation for success in any endeavor, and parenting is no exception. Without confidence we can inadvertently allow the world to dictate our parenting choices, leaving us feeling unsure. We have to shed the weight of conditioning that is cracking our foundation: unworthiness causing guilt, information overshadowing our instincts, and mismanaged stress response.

This requires an *internal* self-improvement project with increased awareness and changing belief systems. We can find inner fulfillment by relying on our own worthiness instead of letting external validation determine our merit. We can determine our values and then apply information instead of letting fear and information dictate our priorities. We can regulate our responses to daily stressors to experience life thriving instead of trudging through life in an exhausted state of survival mode.

Facing your inner wounds can be daunting, but once you feel inner peace, you will be grateful you did the work.

CHAPTER 5
shed the weight of mom guilt

"Comparison is the thief of joy."

-President Theodore Roosevelt

the root of mom guilt

Mom guilt—the heavy weight of inadequacy that plagues modern mothers. It is the sinking feeling we get when we fail to reach unrealistic expectations. It is the nagging voice telling us we are not good enough unless we are doing for others. It is the societal double standards forcing mothers to be caught between "damned if we do but damned if we don't." It is the comparison trap that pulls us into a spiral of shame that steals our internal validation.

Mothers are bombarded with opportunities for self-inflicted "mom-shaming." A social media post of a child's lunch cut into star shapes may cause a mother to feel as if she is failing by cutting her child's sandwich in half with a knife. If a child's friend is on a competitive traveling sports team, the mother may worry her child is missing an opportunity if they do not take part in a similar activity. A mother who works outside the home may feel shame for not making home cooked meals and spending time with her children. When mothers try to rest and relax, it can be hard to ignore the compulsion to do "something productive."

It's as if we are constantly failing to meet invisible benchmarks set for us. Basing our value on factors that we do not control will cause disappointment, regret, and shame. These are stressful feelings that pull our emotional state down, which is why addressing mom guilt is very important for our quality of life. In fact, the term "shame-flammation" refers to the manifestation of negative emotions into inflammation in the body.

How do we heal the modern ailment of mom guilt? As a holistic doctor, my approach to practicing medicine is to solve the cause of the problem producing the symptoms. This is how I approach addressing the stigma of shame that follows mothers; we look for the underlying belief instead of just telling ourselves to not feel guilty.

Where does the belief of mom guilt originate? Let's look at the definition of guilt, which is "being responsible for a specified wrongdoing." Why do women feel they are constantly responsible for wrongdoings? The answer lies deep within our societal conditioning. Elise Loehnen explains in her book *On Our Best Behavior* that "our tradition and culture have decreed that women are inferior."[13] As society's designated "inferior" gender, cultural programming instructs women to *prove* our basic goodness. For instance, when men do something for themselves, the cultural narrative says, "he must need a break." On the other hand, when a woman does something for herself, our culture jumps to judgment. "She shouldn't be resting when there are dirty dishes in the sink. A mother should be spending time with her children. Her poor family won't get a home cooked meal tonight." This double standard has led many women to believe

---

13 Elise Loehnen, *On Our Best Behavior* (New York: The Dial Press, 2022).

our value is based on what we do and how it appears to the world, and not who we are.

So we go through life constantly trying to prove our value through doing, achieving, comparing, and judging. Releasing ourselves of the need to appear flawless will ultimately decrease the burden of mom guilt.

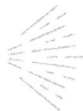 **TO ABSOLVE MOM GUILT, WE HAVE TO SEPARATE OUR WORTH FROM WHAT WE DO OR WHAT OTHERS THINK.**

The path to find our true worth requires us to change directions, to follow our internal compass instead of everyone else's roadmap. This will liberate us from the misdirected shame that is holding our emotional state down.

Let me share an example of my own "mom guilt." On days when I found myself extra busy and tired, I would put together a plate of odds and ends (nowadays referred to as charcuterie) for dinner. I felt guilty for not providing a hot homemade meal because that's what a "good" mom does. However, when I later relayed this regret with my grown daughter, she responded by saying, "Oh, I loved those dinners because it was fun to make it together." Her revelation proves what children truly want is connection, and external expectations may not be in the best interest of our family.

better is okay

Placing our value on results leads to the perfectionism mentality—striving to meet high standards and concern over what others perceive. Many women are caught in this behavior, which is a survival mechanism to avoid disappointing ourselves and others. This is why we keep raising the bar without second guessing the repercussions; we are stuck in autopilot motivated by fear of not measuring up.

It's akin to practicing yoga. Imagine you're barely holding the "pigeon pose," with one leg bent forward and the other leg stretched back. Then the instructor suggests advancing to the "one-legged king pigeon pose," where your arm reaches back and pulls your leg up to your head. You glance around and see someone next to you effortlessly in a one-legged king pigeon pose, and you think to yourself, "Wow, they're better than me. I need to be able to do that to be good at yoga."

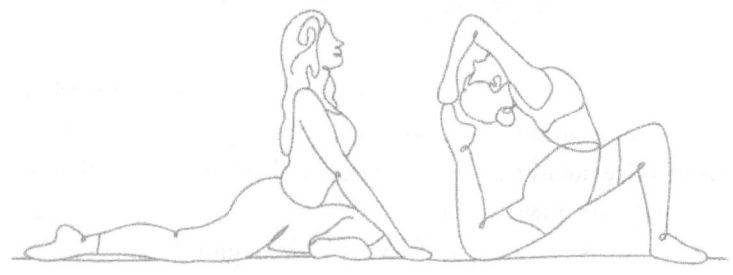

I've noticed mothers falling into the same pattern, constantly pushing themselves to meet the standards of a "good mom." But if we are already unsteady in our current position, how can we keep "advancing the pose"? Yet we can't help but feel like "bad parents" if we choose to stay in the "pigeon pose" instead of striving for the "one-legged king pigeon pose" like everyone else. This pursuit of perfection leaves us flailing, trying to keep up.

Now I'm not saying we shouldn't improve and advance. But let's do it at a pace and level that works for us. Many of us are striving to be better parents than our parents. We shouldn't judge our parents; they did the best they could with the resources they had at the time. Our generation often heard phrases like "big girls don't cry," "I will buy you a new toy if you get all As," or "just eat a can of pasta Os for lunch." It's only natural for us to strive for improvement, and I'm grateful that we are making progress. However, I've witnessed an extreme where parents push themselves to exhaustion, tending to every aspect of their child's emotional, physical, and environmental needs. We may have swung the pendulum too far; it's as if we're overparenting to compensate for any perceived underparenting we might have experienced. We need to find a middle ground and remind ourselves that better is okay. There is so much in between bad and perfect; we can find the sweet spot of not underparenting, but not overparenting.

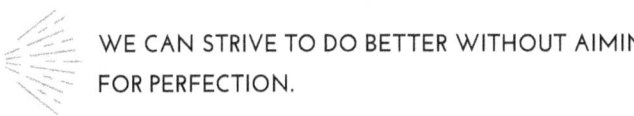
WE CAN STRIVE TO DO BETTER WITHOUT AIMING FOR PERFECTION.

What is better? That is up to you. There is no "right" way to be a mother, just your way. If there was a perfect way to parent, there would only be one parenting book (besides this one, of course). As long as we try our best, we will not fail at parenting. Children are resilient—apart from neglect and abuse, our actions will unlikely make or break them. Surprisingly, children need fundamental elements: connection, unconditional love, and support.

Allow me to reference a study conducted on English survivors of World War II.[14] The government evacuated children from war-torn London to the countryside, but some parents chose to keep their children with them. When comparing the outcomes of these children as adults, those who stayed in the war zone with their parents had better results. While I acknowledge that this situation is complex, it highlights the significance of children's connection to their parents. Truly, all they need is us.

---

14 D. Foster, S. Davies, H. Steele, "The Evacuation of British Children during World War II: A Preliminary Investigation into the Long-Term Psychological Effects," *Aging Ment Health* no. 7 (2003): 398-408, doi: 10.1080/1360786031000150711.

We need to prioritize connection with our children and not allow ourselves to travel down a guilt trip for everything else. This is yet another reason to not overextend ourselves by pursuing the "king pigeon pose" of parenting, while sacrificing our relationship with ourselves and our family.

fear of missing out (fomo) parenting

Modern parenting often leads us to chase external markers of childhood such as rate of development, level of grades, what team they are on, type of school, and ultimately, adult success. This is a pet peeve of mine. If I ask parents how their child is doing, and they reply with a resume—3.9 GPA, two advanced classes, elite baseball team, violin lessons—it is unsettling. The parent is missing the point by defining childhood with these superficial measures.

As George Glass, MD, expertly explains in his book *The Overparenting Epidemic*, "We want the best for them (our children) and fear the worst if we don't pull out all the stops."[15] Parents are worried their child will miss an opportunity that contributes to future success, so they overcompensate and go to extreme measures to appease that worry. I call this FOMO (fear of missing out) parenting—a form of helicopter parenting that is driven by the compulsion to control outcomes. But since we are ultimately *not* in control, we find ourselves flailing in our efforts.

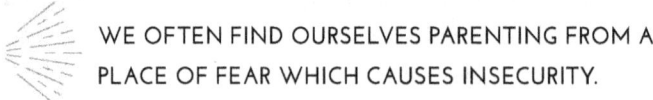

WE OFTEN FIND OURSELVES PARENTING FROM A PLACE OF FEAR WHICH CAUSES INSECURITY.

There are examples of parents intervening even into adult years. When my daughter enrolled in college, I received an email from the school's

---

15 George Glass, MD, and David Tabatsky, *The Overparenting Epidemic: Why Helicopter Parenting Is Bad for Your Child (and Dangerous for You, Too!)* (New York: Skyhorse Publishing, 2022).

administration with helpful information for parents. One paragraph stood out: the school stated a policy that professors will not reply to parents and urged parents to have the student contact teachers about assignments, grade disputes, etc. If they had to make a policy, that means there have been parents contacting professors on behalf of adult college students. These extreme measures illustrate the pressure modern parents feel to interpose in their child's lives.

Comparison amplifies FOMO. Mothers are repeatedly judging themselves, especially with increased access to details of others' lives through modern technology and media. My mother was less aware of how another mother cut her child's sandwich or how many goals her friend's child scored at their last game. If we allow comparison to seep into our daily lives, it can cause ungratefulness, which is the black cloud of feelings. For example, in middle school I recall getting a new pair of black LA Gear high-top tennis shoes that I was thrilled to wear—until I saw a friend with the same shoes in a neon pink color. Suddenly, my "ugly" black pair lost its appeal compared to the "prettier" pink version.

While parenting is undoubtedly more important than the color of tennis shoes (although to a middle schooler, it may feel just as significant), parents can easily fall into this pitfall that is filled with self-doubt and instability. Fear of missing out can truly steal the joy from parenting.

secure and sure (sas) parenting

The opposite of FOMO parenting is what I call SAS (Secure and Sure) parenting. Parenting from a place of security requires a conscious effort to redefine our worth and accept imperfection.

Redefining our value requires us to refocus our priorities on what matters—our family. When feeling guilty about something, ask yourself if it serves the best interest of you and your family. If not, then we should not waste our time worrying. I find this mantra helpful:

MY WORTH AS A MOM COMES FROM MY CONNECTION TO MY FAMILY, AND NOT WHAT I DO.

It's important to decouple our value from our productivity. We have to confront and heal underlying false beliefs to shift our mindset. This process is different for everyone, but the goal is to trace the belief back to the experience that created it. Maybe it was being scolded for not achieving a certain outcome or being praised for being productive but ignored when not. Whatever the case, somewhere along the way we got the message that our worth relies on what we do and not on who we are.

We can replace that belief with a new belief—we are good mothers no matter what we or our children achieve or do not achieve. If we find our child not doing well in school, in a difficult relationship, or otherwise struggling, we can separate ourselves and realize we can only do so much. At the end of the day, they are their own people and not a reflection of our success or failure.

> I will give you an example, from my own mothering journey, of separating my worth from my daughter's outcomes. My daughter made the decision to complete her last two years of high school through an online program from home. This situation tested our merit as parents. Could we still be considered "good" parents if she wasn't associated with a particular school or engaged in traditional extracurricular activities? Well-meaning friends and family expressed concerns about her socialization and questioned what she would be "doing" in terms of sports and activities. However, we held onto the understanding that our internal worth is not defined by external factors, and our inner value and goal was for her to live authentically instead of for external validation.

shed the weight of mom guilt

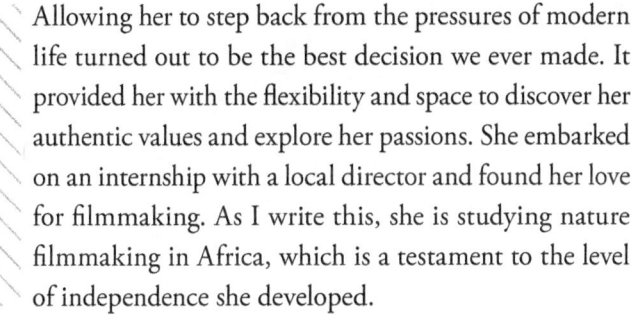 Allowing her to step back from the pressures of modern life turned out to be the best decision we ever made. It provided her with the flexibility and space to discover her authentic values and explore her passions. She embarked on an internship with a local director and found her love for filmmaking. As I write this, she is studying nature filmmaking in Africa, which is a testament to the level of independence she developed.

Embracing imperfection helps build a solid foundation for a peaceful experience. Making mistakes is a part of being human; remember, we are not robots. And of course, make sure the "mistakes" are based on your family's standards, not based on societal standards. One way to accept our flaws is to realize that it is good for us to model our humanness to our children. After all, just like a perfectly clean house is not truly lived in, a perfect life is not truly lived. Many of my family's most memorable moments come from the "comedy of errors" of life.

I know this is easier said than done. In fact, as I am writing a chapter on letting go of perfectionism, I am looking up synonyms and rewriting sentences left and right. My collaborator Liz Wolfe has a phrase to remind herself to relinquish this expectation: F**k It. The laundry is not folded and put away? F**k It—we are using clothes straight from the laundry basket. I burned dinner while multitasking? F**k It—we are ordering takeout. Her daughters have mimicked and created their own mantras (without cursing) to help them accept imperfection.

We can make the transition from FOMO parenting to SAS parenting by absolving ourselves of comparison and perfectionism. Recognizing that we are good people no matter what we do is simple, but not easy. Instead of relying on the outside world to tell us, we need to tell the world: *we are worthy!*

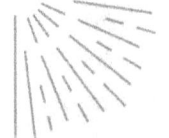

Take Home

CHAPTER 5
shed the weight of mom guilt

◇ **You are worthy.** Your value is not based on what you do or what others think.
- What makes you feel most valued?
- Is that based on your own standards or those of others?
- Next time you feel guilty for something, evaluate if the feeling is based on actual wrongdoing.

◇ **Better is okay.** You can improve without being perfect.
- What do you want to do better than your parents?
- How can you improve?
- Are you swinging the pendulum too far and aiming for perfection? If so, how can you find balance?

◇ **You are not missing out.** Parenting based on comparison and fear will lead to insecurity.
- Do you worry about your child not meeting certain benchmarks?
- Have you acted on this worry to intervene in their life?
- Do you find yourself comparing aspects to others?
- If so, how can you not let comparison affect you?

◇ **You can be secure and sure.** You are a good mother no matter what your child does or does not do.
- Think of an aspect where you connect your value to a result.
- Can you think of an experience that caused that belief? Think of times when you were praised for good results or received negative reinforcement for bad results.
- How can you replace that belief with a truth that your worth is not based on that result?

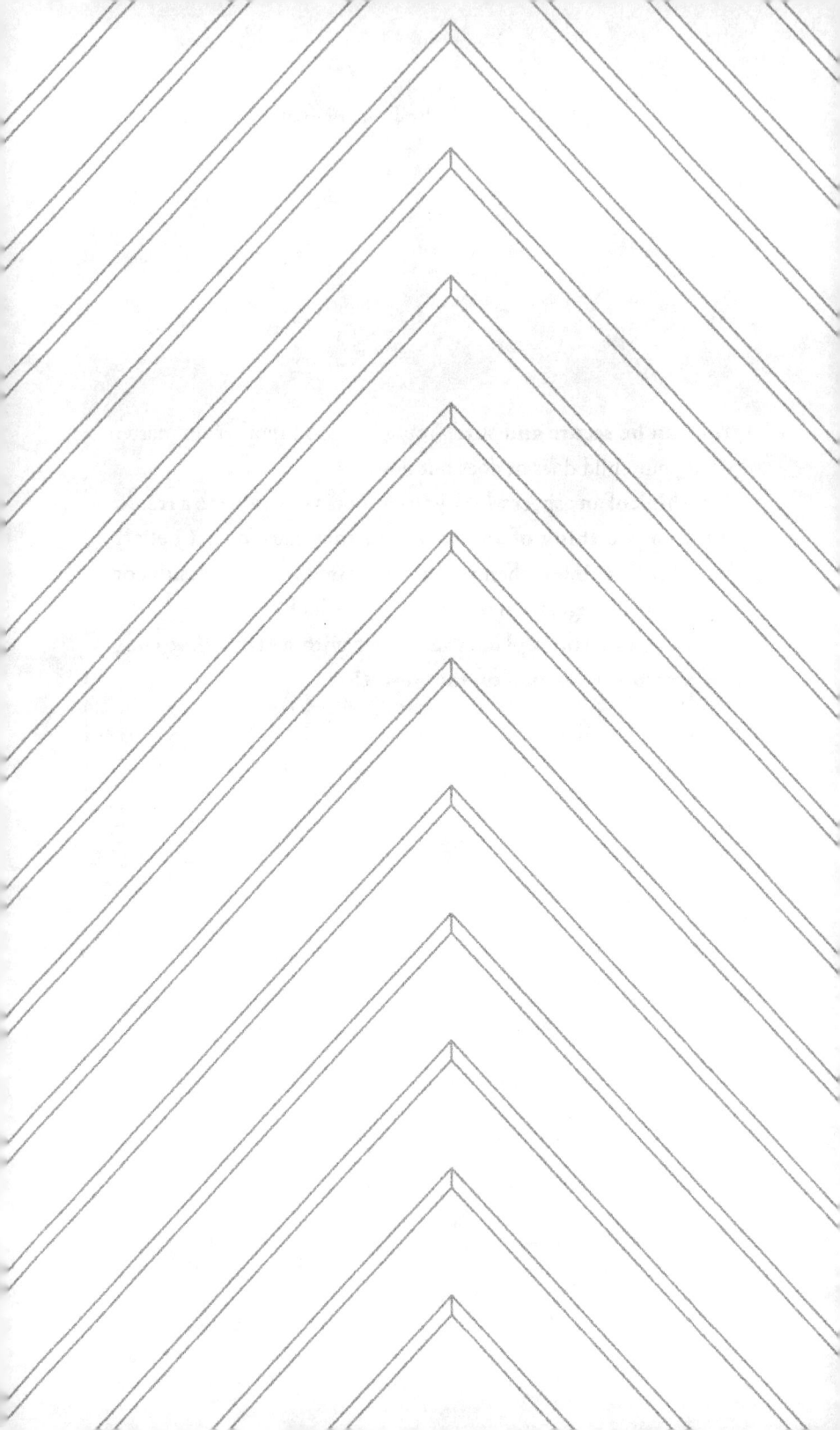

CHAPTER 6
weeding through the information overload

"*Forever tried to find some sort of guidance. But all I need is already here.*"

-"Breathe In," song by Praana

discernment

All right, moms, I do not have to tell you—the information overload these days is no joke. It's like we're drowning in a sea of "do this, but not that," "buy this, not that," and "parent this way, but definitely not that way." I mean, come on, how are we supposed to keep up?

On the one hand, it's amazing that we have all this knowledge at our fingertips. But let's be real, it can also be totally overwhelming. If we're not careful, that blessing of information can quickly turn into a curse.

That's where discernment comes in, my friends. Discernment is the ability to judge and make sense of all this information that is

59

thrown at us—whether it is from well-meaning friends and family, social media's trending mom, or a favorite blogger. I know this is easier said than done. These days, it can be tough to find reliable sources we can trust. Maybe our parents do things differently, or our primary care provider is just too darn busy to give us the guidance we need. But that's where we need to put on our discernment hat and do the legwork ourselves.

But it goes beyond determining the truthfulness of the information; we also have to determine if it is applicable to our lives. We need to do what works for our family, not just what the latest parenting trends say we "should" be doing.

IT'S NOT JUST ABOUT WHETHER THE INFORMATION IS FACTUAL. IT'S ABOUT FIGURING OUT WHAT ALIGNS WITH YOUR VALUES AND GOALS AS A PARENT.

When you can sift through all the noise and figure out what resonates with you, that sense of confidence and clarity is priceless. Embrace your inner discernment ninja and start making decisions that are the best fit for your family.

the forest through the trees

Ah, the age-old dilemma of not missing the forest by focusing on the trees. But it truly applies to the current trap of modern commercialism and access to information. It's easy to get caught up in the latest shiny gadget or information trend, but we must stay focused on the big picture.

I often talk to moms who are convinced they "need" items like a water ionizer for their homes. They have fallen into the rabbit hole of "guidance" from social media, family, or friends. As a result,

weeding through the information overload

these moms feel like their family will "suffer" if they do not have the latest must-have fad. I ask them to discern if that is truly a need and a priority. Now I'm not saying there is a right or wrong thing to do. But you should not miss the more important aspects, such as filtering water, by using resources on minute details such as alkaline versus acidic water.

Getting preoccupied with "keeping up with the Joneses" reminds me of the Aldi's middle aisle phenomenon. For those of you who have not had the pleasure of experiencing this icon, it is the grocery store chain's non-food close-out section—you walk in to buy basic groceries, and you walk out with a food dehydrator, a cardboard cat house, or some other random doodad that you just "had to have." Marketers are experts at making us think we "need" things that we really do not. And unfortunately, that mentality has crept into the world of parenting.

But here's the thing: you're the one in the driver's seat.

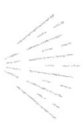 YOU DECIDE HOW YOU'RE GOING TO MOTHER YOUR CHILD, AND THEN YOU FIND THE TOOLS AND RESOURCES TO SUPPORT YOUR DECISIONS, NOT THE OTHER WAY AROUND.

Don't let the latest trends or your neighbor's fancy new baby monitor dictate your parenting approach. Stay true to your values and your vision for your family. Before you jump on the latest parenting product bandwagon, take a step back and ask yourself, "Do I actually have a problem that this would solve? Or am I just getting sucked in by the hype?"

We need to avoid being so caught up in the trees that we miss the whole dang forest. Keep your eye on the big picture—discernment is the key to staying focused on what really matters.

fear is counterproductive

Fear is a powerful motivator, and marketers have become masters at wielding it, especially when it comes to parenting. Our deepest worries often revolve around our children's health and well-being, making us vulnerable targets for scare tactics. These tactics are employed across industries, all in the pursuit of driving sales and compliance.

As a doctor who has stepped away from the conventional medical model, I've seen firsthand how fear can be used to manipulate patients into medical decisions that may not be in the best interest of the individual. And the same holds true in the wellness space, where messages about the dangers of toxins, fast food, and acidic water (I do not have anything against water alkalinizers, they are just a good example) can create an impossible feat for mothers tasked with maintaining a "perfect" lifestyle. I observe mothers who are running themselves in the ground to control their child's diet and environmental exposures, but the immense effort is causing distress. Worrying that our family will suffer from our inaction motivates us to keep toiling at these duties, just like FOMO parenting we discussed previously.

While it may spur us to action in the moment, the resulting stress and anxiety can defeat the purpose.

Remember the mirroring phenomenon—if we are stressed then our children are stressed.

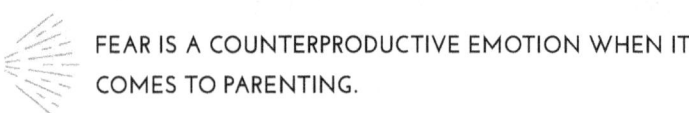

FEAR IS A COUNTERPRODUCTIVE EMOTION WHEN IT COMES TO PARENTING.

It is better to have occasional exposure to fast food or plastic toys if it helps keep your sanity—what is most important is supporting your family's regulation. We can find the equilibrium of making our family's lifestyle the best possible, while also maintaining our sense of selves.

Bottom line: be wary of worry. If you are compelled to do something to pacify anxiety, then question the underlying intentions and follow the money trail. We must strive to make choices that prioritize our family's overall values and needs, without succumbing to the force of fear.

control the helicopter

It's not just the external information we need to discern—we also need to be mindful of the information within our own families. Think about how much things have changed just in the last generation or two. Our parents often followed the motto "no news is good news." They did not have all these constant updates and ways to monitor their children's every move.

But these days? Whew, the amount of information parents have access to is somewhat overwhelming. Nanny cams, online school portals, app trackers, constant communication—it's like we can be privy to every single detail of our kids' lives. And while that might seem like a good thing, the truth is, it can do more harm than good.

If we aren't careful, we can slip into hypervigilance where we don't give our kids the chance to learn on their own. And that's not doing us any favors. I've seen mothers obsessing over homework and grades on their child's school portal on a daily basis, causing discontentment between mom and child. I've seen mothers losing sleep over watching the video monitor of their sleeping baby. I've seen mothers texting their children the whole time they are at a friend's house to get every detail. We need to find ways to take back the controls of our helicopters.

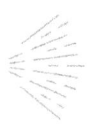

> WE CAN WALK THE TIGHTROPE OF BEING INVOLVED AND ENGAGED, BUT NOT TO THE POINT OF SMOTHERING OUR KIDS AND NOT ALLOWING THEM TO DEVELOP THEIR OWN RESILIENCE.

It's about prioritizing and discerning what information is truly important, and what's just noise that's going to leave us feeling overwhelmed and anxious. Consider checking the school portal once a month, turning the video on the monitor off and just listening for a cry, or waiting to hear about your child's playdate when they get back home.

Our kids need us to be grounded and present, not constantly worrying and micromanaging every aspect of their lives. I tell parents it is like riding a horse—it's the delicate dance of letting go of the reins to let the child have independence, but also pulling back to keep them in check. This counterbalance is one of the most important things we can do as parents.

how to weed

Weeding through the information overload is exactly that—discarding the "weeds" of information and things that do not serve you and your family, while leaving the "flowers" of things that do fit.

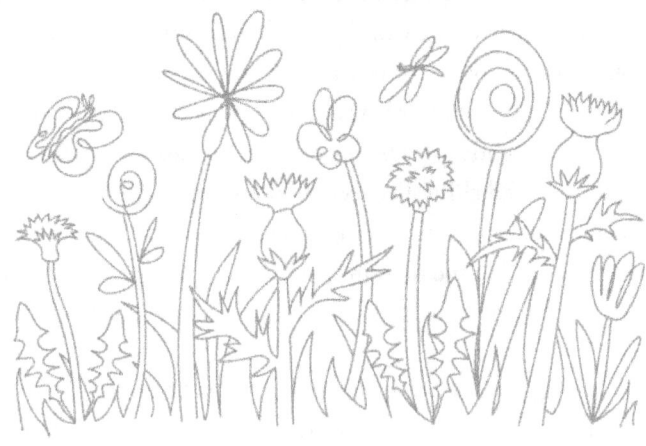

We can start by exploring what "fits." This requires clarity to figure out what are *our* authentic inner values. Then comes the process of alignment—figuring out which information follows what we value. That is how we determine if the plant is a weed or a flower. Remember one person's flower, may be another person's weed, which illustrates the importance of discernment.

Take the example of my patient's mom who was starting to feed her infant solid foods. She was told by a well-meaning friend to mix breastmilk in purees when starting solid foods, and it just wasn't sitting right with her. You know what I told her: there's no "right" way, just her way. It may have worked for the mother who told her that advice, but if it doesn't work for you then it is not a priority. The priority is starting solid foods the way that works for your family.

And that's the secret sauce, my friend. We have to stay true to ourselves and not let the constant barrage of advice make us question our own instincts. Think about our grandmothers—they had less access to information, but they didn't seem to doubt themselves nearly as much as we do these days. And you know why? They trusted their gut and did what felt natural to them. Although there may have been times they should have questioned themselves—such as when giving whiskey to fussy babies!

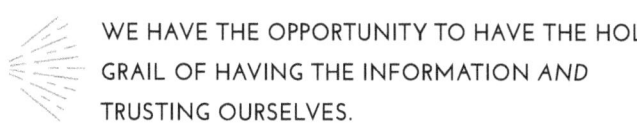

WE HAVE THE OPPORTUNITY TO HAVE THE HOLY GRAIL OF HAVING THE INFORMATION *AND* TRUSTING OURSELVES.

As a parent, you may often find yourself asking, "Is it okay if I do it this way?" And here's where I turn the question back to you. "What do you think?" More often than not, parents seek my "expert opinion" just to validate what they already believe is right. But the only person who truly needs to validate those choices is *you*. We're the experts when it comes to our own families. We know what works best for us, and that's what really matters.

So let's take a deep breath, tune out the noise, and focus on what resonates. Let's be the confident, intuitive parents we were born to be, and not let anyone or anything get in our way.

Take Home

CHAPTER 6
weeding through the information overload

◇ **You can discern.** Be intentional about judging information, actions, or choices. Decide if they align with your and your family's needs, values, and desires.
- Next time you are presented with new information, discern if it is reliable and factual.
- Then listen to your gut feeling to decide if the information resonates with you and your values.

◇ **Focus on priorities.** Do not get lost in the details and miss the big picture.
- Next time you are making a decision, evaluate your priority.
- Are there areas where you expend resources that may not be a priority?

◇ **Avoid fear.** Be aware of being motivated by worry.
- Next time you are prompted to buy or do something, evaluate the motivation.
- When something makes you worry, decide if your concern is valid.

◇ **Control micromanaging.** Find your balance of being involved without hindering your child's independence and resilience.
- **Next time you want to intervene or monitor your child, determine if your motivation is to help them or to help alleviate your worry.**
- **Are there areas where you can decrease your intervention or monitoring of your child?**

◇ **Learn how to discern.** Define and be true to your values and priorities by determining if the information aligns with those.
- **Write down your priorities for you and your family. Next time you are having difficulty discerning information or making a decision, use this list to guide you.**

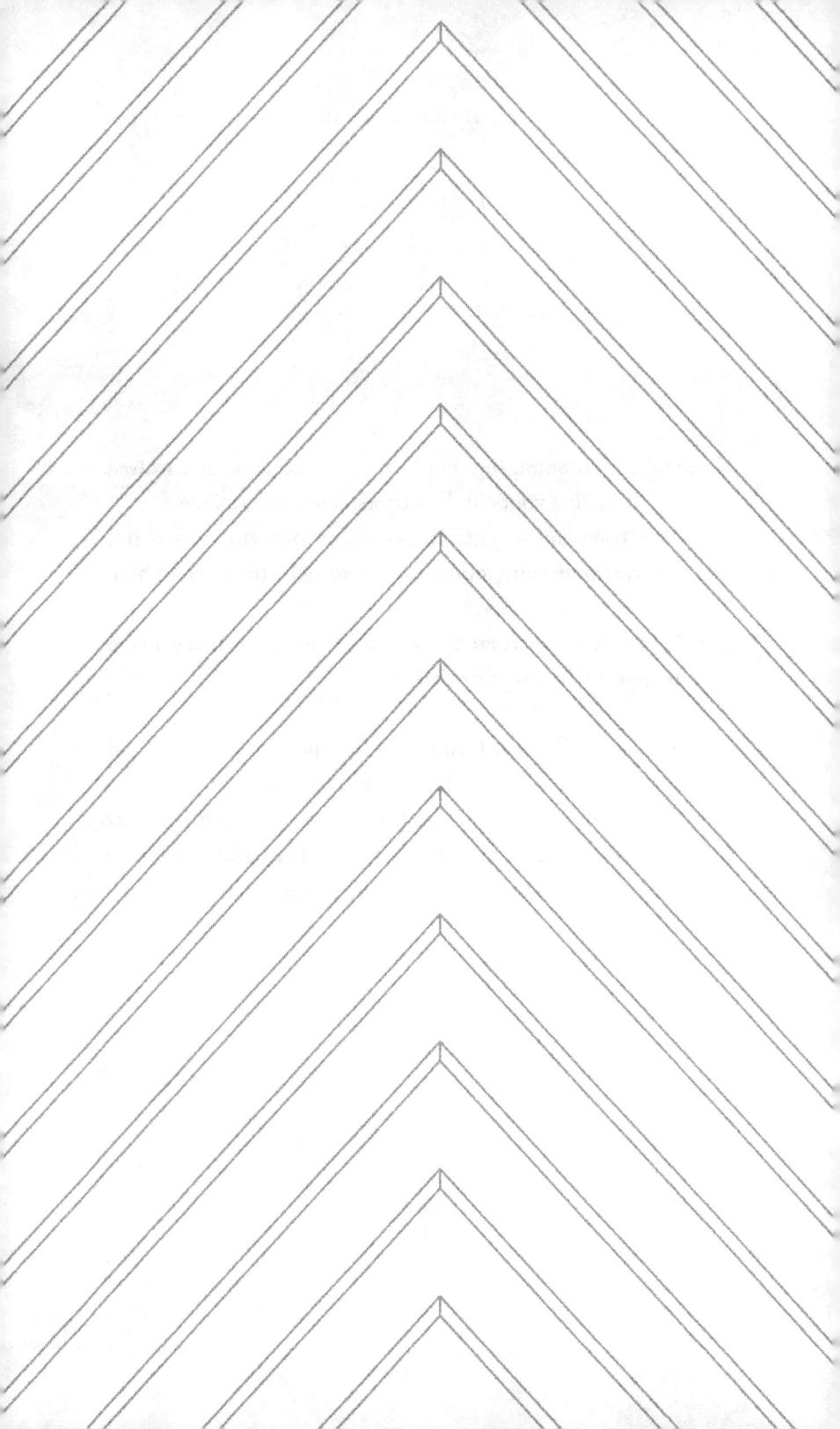

CHAPTER 7

thrive—not just survive

"*The purpose of this glorious life is not simply to endure it, but to soar, stumble, and flourish as you learn to fall in love with existence.*"

-Becca Lee

live to fight another day

During my surgery training, I had a saying for critically ill patients that required full-scale medical measures for survival: keep them alive to fight another day. There are times when motherhood can feel similarly—getting through the day unscathed to be able to do it again the next day. The challenges of raising children can sometimes feel relentless and depleting. As moms, it's all too easy to find ourselves in a perpetual state of merely enduring life without the bandwidth to fully engage with life. And when we're operating from that depleted place, parenting becomes exponentially more challenging and less enjoyable.

It is common to have difficult days, but if we are not careful the days can turn into months, and we can find ourselves in a *prolonged* state of survival. Without reprieve and recuperation, our bodies can develop irritability, insomnia, inability to relax, muscle tension, fatigue, and brain fog (difficulty focusing, making decisions, or remembering). You might be nodding your head in agreement as you read that list of ailments; they are unfortunately far too common in modern mothers.

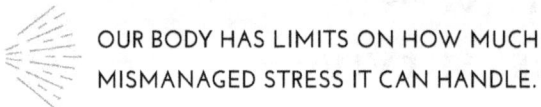

OUR BODY HAS LIMITS ON HOW MUCH MISMANAGED STRESS IT CAN HANDLE.

Even a doctor cannot escape this reality. My body sent me a clear message that it needed a break when I developed a thyroid disorder. Initially, I felt disempowered and frustrated because I thought I was doing everything "right" to be healthy—eating a whole-food diet, exercising, and taking supplements. At the time my only remedy was to double down these efforts to make my diet more strict, increase the supplements, and push myself to exercise more. But instead of making me feel better, those endeavors left me feeling worse. I waved a white flag and admitted defeat that I—a medical doctor with a nutrition degree and training in integrative medicine—could not help myself.

In a fateful turn of events, one of my patient's moms shared her sister's story that led me on my own path to healing; ultimately, it was a patient who helped the doctor. Essentially, her sister found ways to manage her stress response and allow her body the rest it needed to heal itself. That conversation was a revelation for me. I realized that I had been solely fixated on the physical, rather than taking a more holistic, mind-body approach. Learning about nervous system dysregulation explained my symptoms and why my condition worsened when I added more pressure with an intense lifestyle—my body was telling me it needed less stimulation, not more.

stress is not what happens to us

Now I know what you're thinking. *If one more person tells me to "reduce my stress," I'm going to vomit.* I get it. As mothers, we cannot just say, "Sorry, I've reached my allowed amount of stress today; the children will just have to take care of themselves." Or "Oh, the sink is leaking water, but I need to reduce my stress, so I am going to ignore it."

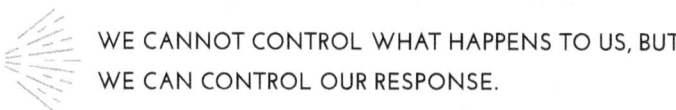

WE CANNOT CONTROL WHAT HAPPENS TO US, BUT WE CAN CONTROL OUR RESPONSE.

Here is an anatomy and physiology lesson to explain how we can manage our mind and body's response to outside stimuli. Our nervous system has two main modes: parasympathetic (rest and repair) and sympathetic (fight or flight). The sympathetic, or "survival mode," is an instinctual, automatic response that originates in the part of our brain called the limbic system. This primitive area is sometimes called the "lizard brain" because we have it in common with reptiles. When these nerves are activated, our bodies respond by flooding our system with cortisol and adrenaline—this is an example of the mind-body connection. These chemical messengers cause our bodily functions to be alert and ready: the brain shifts from logic to reflexes, the lungs breathe fast and shallow, the heart beats faster, the pupils dilate, and the gut slows down to shunt energy to muscles. Evolution created this response as essential to our survival, allowing us to perceive danger and run or fight for our lives.

What was initially a positive trait can become detrimental if left unchecked in today's modern world. Our bodies cannot easily

motherhood makeover

distinguish between a real, immediate threat (like a lion chasing us) and the everyday stressors we perceive (an upsetting text, a leaking sink, or a crying child). What can we do to control our response to these daily disturbances?

Let's go back to our ancestral days for answers. After all, they had real threats such as predators, but they must have handled them because we survived as a species. One would think the stress of a real predator would be more damaging than a text or tantrum. However, there are key reasons modern stress is maladaptive. Cavemen's stressors were tangible—such as the lion—so they were either eaten or escaped into the safety of their den. Their body experienced peaks of stressful events, but then valleys of calm.

In modern times it can be difficult to get repose as our body perceives unrelenting threats. Technology gives constant access to stressors, making it hard to disconnect. Intangible worries such as bills, emails, or deadlines do not "go away" like the lion does, confusing our body into thinking the threat still exists.

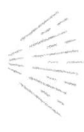 WE HAVE LITTLE ESCAPE IN OUR MODERN CONTEXT; THERE CAN BE CONSTANT INTRUSIONS CAUSING PERSISTENT MID-LEVEL STRESS INSTEAD OF UPS AND DOWNS.

As Kelly Noonan Gores writes in her book *Heal*, "our body's stress response is designed for a sprint—fight or flight to save your life—but these days we are all running a chronic stress marathon."[16]

If we do not allow ourselves to decompress like the cavemen in their cave, then our body assumes there is an emergency and chronic disease may ensue, as my body illustrated. The solution is in the word "dis-ease"; we need to help ourselves become "with ease" after the survival response is no longer needed.

---

16 Kelly Noonan Gores, *Heal* (New York: Atria Books, 2019).

triggered parenting

Beyond physical ailments, a chronic stress response can also be detrimental to our mental health and life experience. Hannah Abad, a certified mindset and resilience coach, uses the analogy of running a marathon with a bear chasing you versus winning a million-dollar prize at the finish line.[17] When we are in a survival state, we are motivated by fear. Our body is running to "protect" us from a threat (the bear). On the other hand, if we are operating from a place of regulation, we can be motivated by rewards (the million dollars). You can imagine the different experience of running towards a million dollars instead of trying not to become a bear's dinner.

The truth is, so many of our challenges have roots in operating from survival mode—we are not our grounded and logical selves. When our lizard brain is active, it inactivates other parts of our brain so we do not overthink as we are fighting for our lives. As the insightful author Hunter Clarke-Fields explains in her book *Raising Good Humans*, "When our brain has mistakenly perceived a threat, the autopilot reactions bypass the prefrontal cortex, and you literally cannot access the rational parts of your brain when the stress response is triggered."[18] Basically, we stop thinking and only react reflexively—after all, if we are running from a lion, our body doesn't want us to stop and contemplate the weather.

Obviously, life threatening events can initiate the survival sequence. But we also have triggers that can push the emergency button of our amygdala. When I explain triggers to others, I tell an unfortunate story

---

17 Liz Wolfe, host, "From Burnout to Breakthrough: Peak Performance Strategies with Hannah Abad," *Balanced Bites*, Episode 466, 12 August 2024. https://realfoodliz.com/balanced-bites-podcast-466-from-burnout-to-breakthrough-peak-performance-strategies-with-hannah-abad/
18 Hunter Clarke-Fields, *Raising Good Humans: A Mindful Guide to Breaking the Cycle of Reactive Parenting and Raising Kind, Confident Kids* (Oakland: New Harbinger Publications, 2019).

about my flock of free-range chickens. At one point, a hawk killed one of my chickens under a tree in our backyard. From that point on, the entire flock avoided that tree, as their brains had encoded it as a site of potential danger. For the chickens, the tree equals death, therefore the tree triggers a survival response to avoid it.

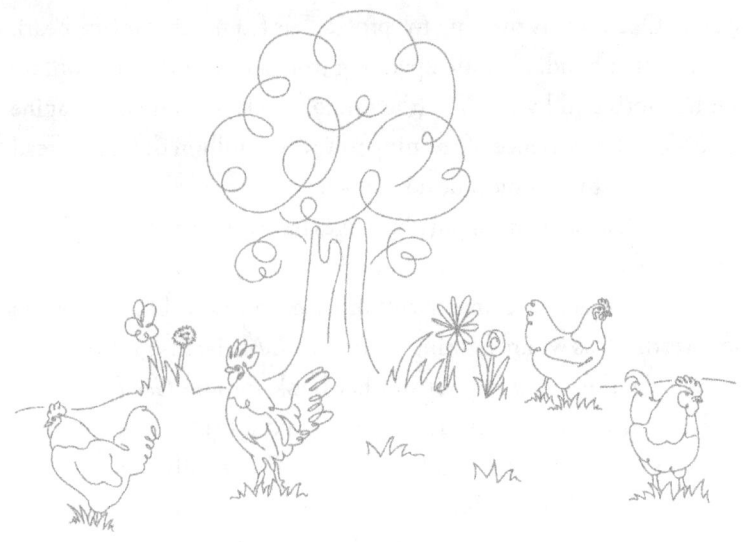

In our modern lives, those triggers can be far more subtle and pervasive such as negative comments on social media or siblings arguing. We can be surrounded by versions of my chicken's tree of death and trapped in our primitive brain. Without rational thinking, it is difficult to differentiate between true alarms requiring our full attention and false triggers that need to be consciously disarmed before they provoke an inappropriate response. Left unchecked, this can create a profoundly negative experience of parenting, one where we're constantly reacting rather than reasoning. Think about a lizard who only has this type of brain; they are always on alert and run at any sudden movement. That does not seem like a peaceful existence.

thrive—not just survive

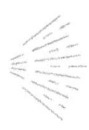
WITHOUT THE SELF-AWARENESS TO RECOGNIZE WHEN WE'RE IN SURVIVAL MODE, WE END UP PARENTING FROM A PLACE OF OVER-REACTIVE AUTOPILOT RATHER THAN A LOGICAL GROUNDED PRESENCE.

Living life through the lens of our amygdala pushes us with *fear* instead of leading us by our true *intentions*. Shifting out of survival mode changes our whole perspective and experience, much like running towards a million dollars instead of from a hungry bear. It helps us be able to show up as our best, most centered selves. And the quality of our interactions, as well as the deeper connections we share, will be profoundly enhanced.

> I remember when my own daughter, who was nineteen at the time, texted me a selfie of her and a rhinoceros while she was on safari in Africa. Luckily, I received that photo *after* I had learned to manage my nervous system's response. The "old me"—the one still stuck in that anxious, survival-driven mentality—would have immediately gone into interrogation mode about the "threat" of the rhino. I would have bombarded her with questions. What were the qualifications of the safari guide? Was she staying alert and careful? Had she considered all the potential risks? I would not have been able to simply be present with her and appreciate her sharing an important experience with me. But the "new me"—the one who had learned to regulate her nervous system and reclaim her rational, prefrontal capacities—was able to approach that situation very differently. I could listen with unbiased interest, trust her judgment, and share in the experience as a caring,

supportive parent, rather than a panicked worrier. We both enjoyed the conversation—she did volunteer the information that the guide had extensive experience, and the animal was a nonaggressive white rhino, which appeased even the logical mommy brain.

how to thrive

As you can see, managing our nervous system is one of the most important things we can do for our well-being and life experience. Unfortunately, emotional intelligence and controlling responses are not a focal point of our society's education or cultural priority. One can argue the opposite—many modern aspects encourage knee-jerk and emotionally driven reactions. Not only are uncontrolled reactions easier, but then modern society promotes quick fixes to alleviate discomfort. Therefore many people turn to unhealthy coping mechanisms, such as substance use and consumerism, to help escape survival mode.

But the good news is we can learn healthy coping mechanisms to regulate, which is the process of controlling and balancing our emotional and physical responses to circumstances at hand. This does not mean being in a state of absolute calm, but rather developing the capacity to skillfully ride the waves of emotion and events. It's okay to not be okay—but it's not okay for us to dwell in one state or another for too long, whether we're stuck in a highly alert, panicky state or a melancholy frozen state. Remember the cavemen; ups and downs are a natural part of life, but the constant living on edge can create an unbalanced life.

How does one balance their nervous system responses? There are two main routes to arriving at a regulated destination. The first is to lay a foundation of calm by addressing past experiences that created the trigger. In our minds, stored negative experiences can create certain beliefs about the world that stimulate an overactive survival center. To disarm this response, we can employ techniques and therapies to dig deeper and unroot the hidden beliefs caused by past experiences. Often, we need the aid of a professional, such as a coach or therapist, to guide the process.

For instance, loud noises are a trigger for my amygdala. You see, I used to be on alert at baseline, but then add a noisy situation, and I would become downright anxious, irritable, and irrational. With the help of a spiritual coach, I was able to trace this trigger back to an accident with fireworks as a child. But it was not the actual experience that created the survival short circuit; it was the inability to express my feelings in that moment due to a lack of support and safety. This created the belief that loud noises are unsafe. To undo that false belief, I had to go back to how it was created, reprocessing the event using inner child visualization and letting myself feel the suppressed emotions. After that process, loud noises are less of a trigger for me. For those of you not familiar with inner child work and healing repressed emotions, the process may sound hokey, but the neuroplasticity of the brain makes it highly effective.

The second route is the day-to-day practice of being attuned to when our survival switch is flipped and helping ourselves turn it back off. Even though working through past experiences can lower our baseline state of mind, we will still experience events that stimulate a stress response. Balancing the mind-body connection is a central focus of the wellness work I do with parents, helping them recognize when they've slipped into that reactionary survival mode, and then equipping them with tools to shift back into a state of calm, parasympathetic mind.

Awareness is the most important step to realize when we are acting reflexively. This can be difficult; after all, we are not thinking logically in that state. Once again, creating time for yourself will allow you to pay more attention to your body and reactions. The more time you spend in a regulated state, the easier it will be to recognize when you are in the survival state.

 TO REGULATE OURSELVES, WE NEED TO BE AWARE OF WHEN WE ARE OPERATING FROM A SURVIVAL RESPONSE, CONTROL OUR RESPONSE, AND GUIDE OURSELVES BACK INTO A BASELINE STATE.

For example, when a toddler throws a tantrum, their amygdala is switched on, and they are like a caged animal fighting to survive. We may even say "they lost it" when describing the incident, which implies that the child was out of control. You cannot reason with a screaming toddler—the best thing is to be available, prevent damage, and help them back down into a rational state. As adults we can have our own type of tantrums—we may not throw ourselves on the ground in the middle of the store, but we can have illogical reactions at times. The best thing we can do is to control the damage and come back down.

Adjusting back to baseline is different for every person and situation. Most of the time just telling your body to "calm down" may not work, and we need to have healthy coping skills in our back pocket to pull out when needed. For some, that might mean deep breathing exercises. For others, it could be taking a physical break, immersing themselves in soothing aromatherapy, or engaging in energizing movement. (I call these "mommy time outs.") Simply recognizing the need to protect our attention—to not feel compelled to respond instantly to every text or email—can go a long way. And in many cases, squelching the overwhelm by reminding ourselves to take it one day (and sometimes one minute) at a time.

Of course, regulation is an ongoing practice, not a one-and-done solution. There will always be moments when our primal responses start hijacking our rational minds, whether due to a major life event or just the normal ups and downs of life. No one is perfect, not even mothers. In fact, as I was writing this chapter, my daughter asked a financial question while I was grappling with unexpected expenses. The timing flipped my survival switch to give an irrational response (and prompted me to put this part in the book). I "lost it," but recognizing I was not in my logical state of mind, I stepped away for a deep breath, then apologized. After all, others are not responsible for triggering us; we are responsible for our reactions.

Our job isn't just to get through the challenges of motherhood, but to actively cultivate a state of resilience and thriving, and ultimately enjoy the experience. Remember that our nervous system is not our enemy but a powerful ally when we learn to work with it. The path to serenity isn't always easy, but it is absolutely within reach.

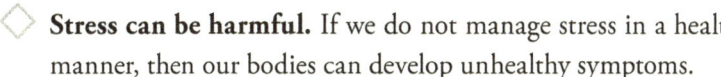

Take Home

CHAPTER 7

thrive—not just survive

 **Stress can be harmful.** If we do not manage stress in a healthy manner, then our bodies can develop unhealthy symptoms.
- Do you have any of these symptoms: irritability, insomnia, inability to relax, muscle tension, fatigue, and brain fog (difficulty focusing, making decisions, or remembering)?

- If so, start noticing how they fluctuate based on different factors: the events of the day, how much time you had for self-care, etc.
- Try to listen to what your body is trying to tell you. If something makes the symptoms worse or better, find ways to decrease or increase those cause and effects.

◇ **Don't persist in survival mode.** Our nervous system stimulation can cause body responses that can be harmful if we do not intentionally give ourselves breaks.
- Next time you are in a stressful situation, take note of your body's response and ability to think logically.
- When the stressful situation is over, take note if your body's and mind's response has calmed or stayed in the alert state.

◇ **Notice triggered responses.** Be aware of situations that cause a survival response.
- What situations commonly "stress you out"?
- Why might those situations be triggers for you?
- How can you manage your response to that situation?

◇ **Develop regulated responses.** Find ways to manage your response to events.
- Next time your stress response is triggered, take inventory of your feelings and how your body is responding.
- Use tools to get your body back into a calm mode.
- How does your body feel and how do you think in calm mode?

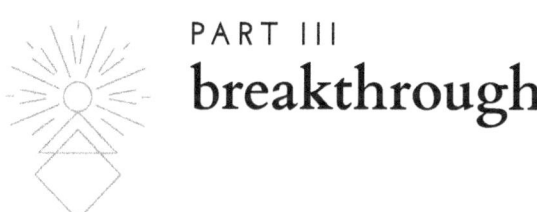

PART III
breakthrough

"Yesterday is not ours to recover, but tomorrow is ours to win or lose."
-Lyndon B. Johnson

ALL RIGHT, MAMAS, let's get real—you've got a lot working against you. The external demands, the inner critic, the swirling emotions—it can feel like an endless obstacle course standing between you and the kind of motherhood you truly desire. But you know what? Mothers are experts at doing hard things. And you are no exception.

You can jump those hurdles. You can break through those barriers. When a mother sets her mind to it, there's no stopping her.

So let's put it all together. Let's take everything we've explored so far—the importance of emotional regulation, the power of self-care, the wisdom in slowing down—and use it to makeover your motherhood and transform the way you show up, not just for your little ones, but for yourself.

This is your breakthrough moment. The chance to leave behind the stress, the burnout, the anxiety and come home to a more balanced, joyful, and *resilient* way of parenting. The path may not be easy, but with the right tools and mindset, I truly believe an authentic life is within your reach. The finish line is in sight. Time to sprint towards the motherhood you know, deep down, you were made for.

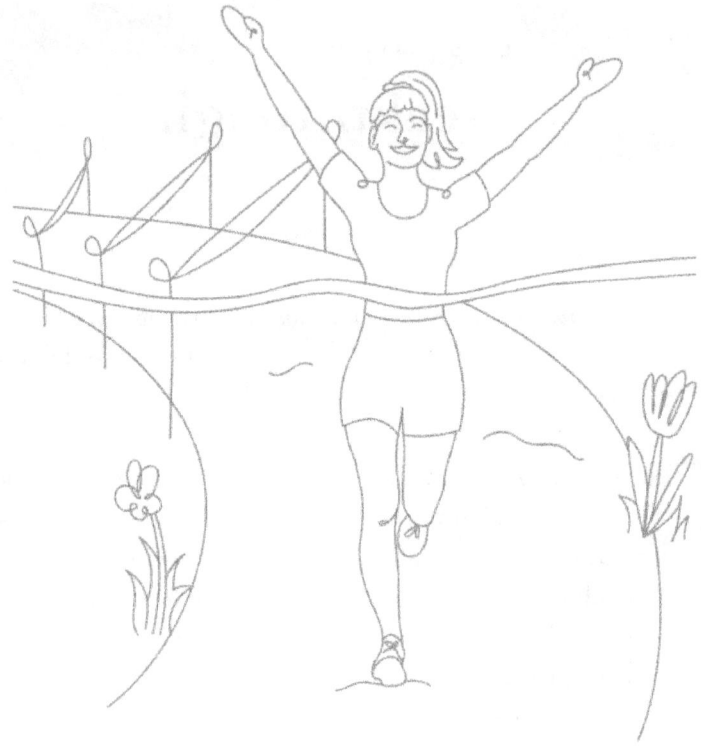

CHAPTER 8
discover your intuition

"Intuition is the intelligence of the heart and the knowledge of the soul. Trust it, and the reason will follow with time."

-Doe Zantamata

mother's sixth sense

Have you ever had the feeling that something was amiss without knowing the details? Or had the urge to make a particular decision but cannot explain why? Call it our sixth sense, our subconscious voice, our gut instinct; they are part of the same phenomenon—our intuition. Intuition may sound like an abstract and far out concept, but it is basically our innate ability to sense beyond our five senses, react using our subconscious mind, and listen to our gut-brain sensory system.

Many people experience a sixth sense beyond hearing, sight, smell, taste, and touch. It is often depicted in religions as faith, the holy spirit, or messages from a higher power. Spiritually speaking, it is the intangible ability to detect energy and emotions. When it comes to mothers, this feeling is our survival instinct in action—the same primal force that allows wild animals to raise healthy offspring without the aid of books or experts. The profound bond between mother and child allows us to sense their needs, their struggles, their joy. I experienced this even from continents away when my daughter was in Africa. There were times when I had a hunch she was dealing with something, then I would get a message confirming she had good or bad news. We can tap into this sense to help guide us in caring for our children.

Let's delve into the idea of conscious versus subconscious, which clarifies the concept of intuition. Our conscious mind is the part of our brain that uses logical thinking that we can explain rationally, such as making a decision based on the pros versus cons. This is just the tip of the iceberg of our complex mind. There is something deeper: our subconscious. While we are mostly aware of our conscious mind, the subconscious is more hidden and automatically draws from our values, beliefs, emotions, habits, and yes, that keen intuitive wisdom passed down through generations. This part of intuition is the ability to understand without the need for conscious reasoning. If you have ever said, "I don't know how I know, but I just know," you were referring to intuition.

Another part that contributes to our intuition is gut instinct, which is just that—our gastrointestinal tract is a part of our sensory system that is surveying our environment. This is considered a kind of "second brain," with the same complex chemistry and neural wiring as the one housed in our skulls. And it is this gut-brain axis that sends signals to alert us when it senses something amiss—the so-called "butterflies in our stomach." Most of the time we may not even recognize this impulse, but it is there trying to tell us something.

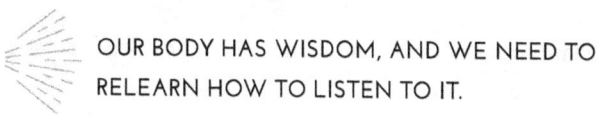 OUR BODY HAS WISDOM, AND WE NEED TO RELEARN HOW TO LISTEN TO IT.

Unfortunately, the current fast-paced and materialistic culture does not understand the nurturing language of mothers; consequently, we've been conditioned to silence and not trust our voice. Societal structures pressure us to ignore our instinct and hand over our decision-making to outside authorities. I have witnessed too many examples of this. Medical providers told parents that "everything is fine" when something inside alerted them there was more going on with their children—and I confirmed their suspicions during a consultation. Mothers are constrained to follow a school's policy even though it contradicts their desires—one of my clients was even told not to hug her child goodbye during drop-off time. How many of us have had similar battles?

No more. It's time to reclaim that intuitive wisdom, stop deferring to external "experts," and start listening to the clarity that resides within. Our motherly intuition is a sacred gift—one that, when honored, can guide us towards the most authentic motherhood journey.

find your path to authenticity

Have you ever had a job that went against your purpose? It can be frustrating and require additional effort. But if you feel your "heart is in it," even the same amount of effort is more fulfilling. You may hardly notice how hard you're working. Parenting can evoke those same feelings. When we are not mothering the way we truly want to, fighting our inner intuition uses extra energy. But if we embrace our values, then the clouds part and the sun comes out in a glorious "aha" moment:

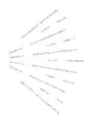 PARENTING IS HARD, BUT IF WE ALIGN WITH OUR AUTHENTIC TRUTHS THEN IT CAN FEEL LESS HARD.

How do we reclaim our own authentic truth? First, we need to tune out the outside noise as we learned to do in Part I—Overcome Forces Working against You. Then we can hear our inner voice and listen to it. The path to honoring your true self is an intentional process involving clarity of your values and alignment of those values to your life.

Clarity involves the subconscious mind, which takes into consideration emotions, values, beliefs, experiences, and instincts. To listen to that part of our mind requires quieting the conscious "thinking" part. It involves taking the time to shut out the outside world and turn internally. This is why spiritual retreats are so powerful; they take us away from our day to day so we can reflect.

Once we clear the noise and uncover our truths, we can begin to apply them to lives. Start by noting when you are working against your values. Find ways to reconcile those more towards your authentic way. For instance, I once spent a day on the beach journaling values and how my life goes against those. I came home and made shifts to bring my reality closer to my desires. One of these values is time outdoors away from technology, but the need to have my phone for patient calls worked against this. Therefore I set a boundary of not taking patient phone calls on the weekend, and now I can disconnect from the phone and connect with nature more.

> One mother's transformation stands out. I first met her while she was a nurse in a large hospital's newborn nursery where I also worked. She was following all of society's "rules" and doing all the typical modern things, but she felt unfulfilled, unsure, and depleted. Later, when I started my own practice, she enrolled her children as patients. That was the start of her journey towards alignment. She made steps to simplify and make space to align her and her family's life. Whenever I would see her at her child's next appointment, I would get snippets of the changes.

One time she told me she quit her nursing job and became a mom/baby yoga instructor. Another time she updated me about moving from their modern suburban home to an older home with land. Throughout I witnessed the metamorphosis as her life became more in sync with her truth. She grew from an anxious and less fulfilled mother to a confident and peaceful presence.

If we taught parents the importance of clarity and alignment, we would have much less frustration. It is alarming to me how the process of parenting is given so little priority in our culture. Instead of a baby shower giving mothers physical items to use for the baby, we should give her a sacred retreat where she can clarify her values *before* the baby arrives. Still, it's never too late to listen to your authentic self and reconcile your motherhood.

There is a caution when finding our authentic voice: our subconscious mind can get imprinted with unresolved emotions and events that short circuit our survival response, as we discussed in chapter 7. You need discernment to determine if your instinct is based on your authentic self or a false alarm from your past. Tuning into our nervous system will determine if the impulse is from our survival or intuitive mind. Reactions based on the past are often fearful or stimulating, whereas our true voice should create a sense of peace. When we slow down and listen, our body will tell us all we need to know.

parenting is a multiple-choice exam

When it comes down to it, parenting is a series of decisions—from the first plans during pregnancy to the last decisions of adolescence. At each fork in the road, we make the best decision possible with the information we have at the time. But oh, how our minds can get so easily tangled up in all the options before us!

Let me give you a method I learned when I was studying for the medical school entrance exam. The test prep course taught us to read the question, and before even looking at the multiple-choice answers, to think what we believed the answer to be. Then when we read the choices, if our pre-thought answer was listed, we were advised to choose that one without second-guessing ourselves. You know what? It worked wonders. Those multiple-choice options can really throw us off, with two answers that seem so closely related. But if you trust your intuition first, you're much more likely to land on your best answer. The same principle applies to motherhood.

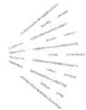 **WHEN YOU'RE FACED WITH A DECISION, TRY TO FIND THE ANSWER WITHIN YOURSELF BEFORE THE OUTSIDE WORLD MUDDIES THE WATERS.**

Do not compromise your values to fit an outside agenda, whether it is how to educate, medical interventions, diet, discipline—the list goes on and on. Make your authentic decision, and you'll start to build that valuable correlation between your intuition and positive results.

Many times, when a parent is grappling with a decision, things will turn out just fine either way. In fact, if there truly is no "wrong" way, then we might as well side with our inner voice and inner values. Then at least you can feel secure in your choice without constant doubt. It takes practice, but I have faith in you. Your inner wisdom knows the way.

Take Home

CHAPTER 8
discover your intuition

◇ **Intuition is instinctual.** We have a sixth sense, gut feeling, and subconscious mind that goes beyond logical reasoning and considers values, beliefs, and instinct.
- **Pay attention the next time you have an inner feeling about something.**
- **Can you determine if that feeling originates from your sixth sense, subconscious, or gut instinct?**

◇ **Seek clarity and alignment.** Clarifying your values and aligning them with your choices can create a more peaceful and fulfilling life.
- **Make a list of your top five values.**
- **List some ways your life and decisions go against those values.**
- **Find three ways you can get your life and decisions closer to your values.**

◇ **Practice making value-led decisions.** Try to make decisions based on your authentic truths to create security.
- **Next time you have a decision to make, think of the choice that you are drawn to before reasoning or rationalizing.**
- **Are you realistically able to go with that choice?**
- **If you are worried about the outcomes for your child, are your concerns valid or invalid?**

CHAPTER 9
build your village

"I would rather walk with a friend in the dark, than alone in the light."

-Helen Keller

where has our village gone?

We all know taking care of a family takes a village, but where has the village gone? I'm not talking about a group of buildings, but a support system—a network of family and friends in the trenches with you, helping with parenting's ups and downs.

In ancestral times, multigenerational families would stay together, which meant multiple women were in proximity and could help each other. They provided not only physical support to share the load of everyday tasks and work, but also emotional and spiritual support. They knew each other, helped in times of need, shared in times of joy, and gave a sense of belonging and security.

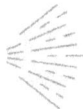 **WITHOUT A SUPPORT SYSTEM, MOTHERS ARE LEFT BEARING THE HUGE BURDEN OF BEING THE WHOLE VILLAGE BY THEMSELVES.**

It's an instinctual impulse to not be alone—lone women and children have lower survival rates in the wild. That's why humans lived in groups in the first place. When we feel alone, it's uncomfortable and unsettling, like a lone wolf. Community helps co-regulate us and gives a sense of safety. If you've ever been to a festival or other group event and felt a positive sense of inclusivity and belonging, that's part of this instinctive feeling. The company of others can help fill our cup. Failing to meet this need can have many consequences, from physical illness like hormone imbalances due to exhaustion, to mental illness like anxiety and depression from lack of emotional support and a sense of belonging.

The events of 2020 shed light on how isolation affected mothers. Rates of mental illness skyrocketed, and I witnessed it firsthand with my patients. I noticed a high level of self-doubt, overparenting, stress, and worry. Mothers had no outlet or connection to process their emotions and difficulties. At the time, I was struggling too, unable to meet a friend for coffee to vent and connect or receive a hug to ease the emotional toll (hugging is one of the best things we can do for our health, as it helps our nervous system calm and releases positive hormones). This was a wake-up call for me, I felt the pain of my "missing" village.

Many of us try to replace the village with a virtual community. Technology has created an interesting situation; while we may not be physically close to a small group of women, we're now exposed to a larger network online. Virtual connection has pros and cons. It has opened up new opportunities to share information and experiences with others; however, we may still feel isolated and crave physical connection. Plus, virtual communication is not as effective, and there's more propensity for bias and marginalization. While virtual connection can be helpful, it can't fully replace physical connection.

While the village of our ancestors may be long gone, the need for community and support remains deeply rooted in our human nature. I asked my daughter's friend, who spent time growing up in a traditional village in Botswana, about his experiences. He confirmed it is efficacious to have a group of people supporting you; at the same time, those villages' lack of modern conveniences make daily life more difficult. During his time in America, he noted the opposite: individualism and lack of community support, but more access to modern conveniences. In our quest for convenience, we have lost our village. What if we could find a way to have the best of both worlds—the benefits of modernism *and* a supportive community?

As mothers, we must be intentional about rebuilding that sense of connection and shared experience. By creating our own supportive community, we can regain the sense of belonging, security, and shared load that our foremothers once enjoyed. It's time to reclaim the village and rediscover the strength that comes from walking this journey together, not alone.

girl talk is important

Have you ever walked away from a girls' night or coffee with a friend feeling refreshed, seen, or like someone "gets" what you're going through? There's a reason for that. Women are more expressive with their emotions as a way to cope, which includes sharing the emotional experience with others. Emotions are, like the term says, "energy in *motion*." If you have ever used the expression "good vibes," that literally means vibrations, which is a form of energy. When we feel an emotion, that is a form of energy. If we do nothing with the energy, it can manifest in physical damage to our body. This is why women need each other emotionally—to express emotions to help regulate and process. We all need our own motherhood support group.

One of the best ways my friends support each other is by keeping it real—we share our true struggles and stories of family life without the sugar-coating. I call my friends my therapists because having a village with whom you can share the ups and downs of motherhood with can be very therapeutic. When I confide in a friend who responds with "I get it," and I know they truly relate, it makes the hardship feel less of a mountain and more of a hill. And when they divulge a situation they are facing, it's comforting that I'm not the only one. Whether it's the toddler demanding to drink from the blue cup that is missing, the dog vomiting on the carpet, partners upset after a stressful day at work, or a burnt dinner because you tended to all the above, knowing we all deal with the same challenges validates our own experiences. And seeing others making it work reassures us that we can too. I always feel lighter and energized after talking with my motherhood support group. It turns out girl talk is an important coping mechanism.

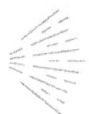 WE NEED OTHERS WHO CAN RELATE TO EVENTS AND HELP US REGULATE EMOTIONS.

On the flip side, sharing positive experiences with others we care about also improves our well-being. It reinforces gratefulness, which is one of the best emotions we can have. Friends truly make the good times better and the hard times feel less difficult.

we aren't meant to do it all

Another reason to have a village is cooperation—we simply aren't meant to do it all ourselves. We were meant to have extended family, friends, and village support. And remember wisdom from the previous chapters—do not succumb to the self-sacrifice narrative, unrealistic expectations, or mom guilt. You are *not* less of a mother if you don't do it all yourself. It makes you a better mother because

build your village

you can use that energy to improve connection with yourself and your children.

Picture this in an extended family home: while mom is feeding the baby, an aunt is watching the older kids, and an elder is making dinner. Now, picture a modern single-family home: the mother is feeding the baby, trying to entertain the older child, and making dinner all on her own. Can you sense the difference and feel why mothers are struggling? No wonder! It's not just the physical struggle, but the mental and emotional toll as well. An inability to do all the things the village used to handle adds to feelings of inadequacy because we constantly feel like it's our fault we are struggling to keep up.

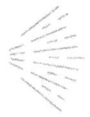 WE ARE NOT FAILING; IT'S THE LACK OF A SUPPORT SYSTEM THAT IS FAILING US.

My dream is to start a self-sustaining community that functions like an actual village with cooperative members helping each other. But even in modern day living, we can find ways to build our own villages so we aren't doing "all the things" by ourselves. Whether it's ride sharing with neighbors, partners helping with tasks, older children playing with friends in the neighborhood, or family watching the kids while you get "me" time—we can find ways to call in reinforcements.

For example, I have a client who has three young kids and runs her own business, yet she's found a way to keep herself at peace. She credits a big part of her peacefulness to a group of four mothers in her neighborhood who have become each other's village. They carpool, rotate playdates, help make meals if someone is going through a tough time, support each other emotionally, and provide stability and security. What a wonderful blessing and a great solution to our modern mothering problems.

Whatever your village looks like, just make sure you have people you can count on to share the load of responsibilities. We aren't meant to do it all alone; embracing cooperation and community is an essential component to our well-being.

the right village

It's not just about having people in our lives—it's about having the right kind of people. Quality matters more than quantity when it comes to our village. Make sure the people in your village are reliable and contribute as much as you do, especially with the limited time and energy mothers have. Nothing is worse than having a village that drains us more than it fills us up. We should use discernment in every aspect of our lives, including our relationships.

Having others who share your values can be incredibly helpful, especially if you're doing things differently than the mainstream. If you're reading this book, chances are you're bucking some modern trends. Having people in the same boat going the same direction can make the journey feel a lot less lonely and give you the power to keep going.

At the same time, it's important to watch out for becoming too polarized or getting stuck in a "mob mentality." All-or-nothing parenting philosophies can increase stress, anxiety, and isolation. It's great to have like-minded friends, but it's also okay to have family and friends with different views, as long as there's mutual respect. Having a variety of perspectives can strengthen our village. The balance is vital—stay functional, not fanatical.

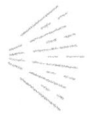

BUILDING A VILLAGE REQUIRES CAREFUL SELECTION, CONTINUAL MAINTENANCE, AND OCCASIONAL REMODELING.

The irony is we're often in the busiest seasons of life when we need a support system the most. Commit to building community into your daily life—make the time to get out there and start building connections. Go to an event you enjoy, join a mother's group, strike up a conversation at the soccer game. The effort is worth it—a thriving village will give you benefits far beyond what you put in.

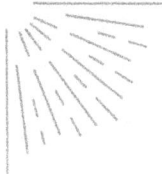

Take Home

CHAPTER 9
build your village

◇ **Mothers need a support system.** You are not meant to be alone; you are meant to have others support you.
- What is your current support system?
- Do you feel adequately supported?
- If you do not have an adequate support system, how can you expand?

◇ **Mothers need emotional support.** Having others to validate and process events and emotions helps regulate yourself.
- When you are having a difficult time, who helps you relate and regulate?
- Can you improve how you use support during difficult times?

◇ **Mothers need physical support.** A mother is not meant to do all the work alone. We need others to share the burden.
- Who do you have that helps share the workload?
- How can you decrease your workload and share it with others?

◇ **Build the right village.** Creating and maintaining a support system takes effort that is worth it. Make space for yourself to focus on your village.
- **Are there parts of your support system that are not serving you well? If so, how can you change that?**
- **How can you make space to expand or maintain your support system?**

CHAPTER 10
improve your well-being

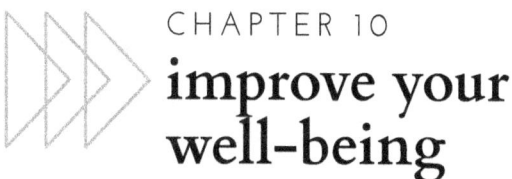

"No matter how much it gets abused, the body can restore balance. The first rule is to stop interfering with nature."

-Deepak Chopra

self-love

Self-care has become a buzzword. It has been depicted as mothers taking care of their basic needs like drinking water, eating, and going to the bathroom. Or represented as giving ourselves "treats" like a bath with aromatherapy or an iced coffee with whipped cream and sprinkles. While such things could be a part of self-care, it's more than that. It is self-love—a way of living that allows you to care for your mind, body, and spirit. It's a *lifestyle* that prioritizes your needs. That may mean taking a break when you are overwhelmed, allowing yourself to cry when you need to, saying no when you don't want to do something, or having a slow-paced morning. Looking after ourselves isn't just some fancy idea—it's something we actively do to show ourselves that our needs matter. Our body listens to our thoughts and actions; our reality becomes what we create.

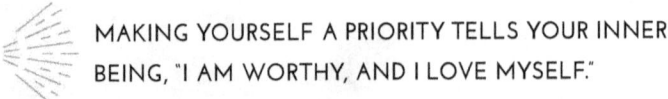
MAKING YOURSELF A PRIORITY TELLS YOUR INNER BEING, "I AM WORTHY, AND I LOVE MYSELF."

Carving out time for ourselves requires taking intentional actions; just like cutting into wood, it requires effort. For instance, one of my favorite simple pleasures is having a slow-paced morning to enjoy a cut grapefruit and drink a mug of tea, so I make it non-negotiable to have at least one morning each week without a time restraint. My family knows to allow my morning ritual or else I will be a disgruntled mama bear. To keep this promise to myself, I've missed activities and outings, but it was worth it for sacred "me" time. (Yes, we can give ourselves permission to not be at every event.) So, what is one of your favorite things, and how can you carve it into your family tree? How can you be proactive and self-advocate for your needs?

When I work with my wellness clients on taking care of themselves, I focus on the basics that contribute to their overall well-being. And I do mean the simple basics, because if we make self-care complicated or stressful, then that defeats the purpose. Focus on health habits like a quality sleep routine, tools for managing stress, nourishing ourselves with nutritious foods and supplements, getting outdoor time, and moving our bodies.

I also emphasize the importance of nurturing our emotional state, like letting ourselves feel our feelings, calm breathing, doing things that make us happy, and having supportive people in your life. Engaging in activities that bring us joy and fulfillment is crucial. It could be painting, writing, gardening, or anything that sparks our passion. The more we improve our inner resilience, the less we have to control the outside.

▷ **cultivate equilibrium**

The first step to improving how we care for ourselves is to make space. As we discussed in previous chapters, there are ways to meet your personal needs *and* your family's needs. This is an ongoing juggling act that can change depending on the events of our lives. I try not to use the word balance, because let's be realistic, there are days when your family needs you less or more.

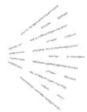 WE SHOULD AIM FOR EQUILIBRIUM—KEEPING OURSELVES WELL INSIDE DESPITE WHAT IS HAPPENING OUTSIDE.

In medical terms, equilibrium means the body keeps internal processes functioning (heart beating, lungs breathing, blood pH normalized), despite external conditions (running a marathon, extreme weather, sitting through a kindergarten choir concert). This can be applied to motherhood—we keep ourselves functional human beings while tending to the chaos that comes with raising tiny humans. Always remember, the glass isn't half empty or half full—it's refillable. Make sure to give yourself free refills of self-love.

Cultivating equilibrium is a continual process of caring for ourselves, whatever that means at any given moment. It's important to remember that meeting our needs can change. At times our bodies might want to go for a run outside, while other times we just need a break to relax and do nothing. It's about listening to what our bodies are telling us and giving ourselves what we need.

One barrier mothers often encounter is that taking care of ourselves becomes another thing on our never-ending to-do list. There is a solution to that dilemma, and that is why I taught you to make space for yourself first. If you've filled up your dinner plate but then notice your favorite food, you cannot add to your plate without taking something off first. You should treat life the same—declutter your time and energy before adding something that takes more. One way of filling your cup is to let less of it get drained out. Remember, if you simplify your motherhood, you will need less "extra" self-love to fill back up.

Another hack is to add self-love into your daily routine. America has taken wellness habits out of our daily lives; consequently, we have to "make time" for exercise, outdoor time, mindful moments, etc. When I visit other countries, I notice how their daily lives have healthy routines built in: walking instead of driving, enjoying meals and other events outdoors, taking longer breaks in the workday instead of succumbing to high demand work environments. But you can find ways to put fulfillment of your needs back into daily life. For instance, I try to take a lunch break outdoors when possible. I get time outside, a break from technology, and nourishment.

tools for the trenches

As mamas, words only go so far; we need actions. That's why it's so important to have a personalized toolkit of tricks and habits that help us keep our cool, even when the chaos of motherhood feels like too much. Think of it like stocking up your arsenal—you need different ammo for different battles. Some days it might be deep breathing exercises and soothing essential oils. Other times, it could be cranking up the tunes for an impromptu kitchen dance party or sneaking in a quick workout. We need to have those go-to tools readily available, so you can easily reach for what you need in the moment.

My toolbox includes little "self-care stations" I set up around my home. For me, that looks like having healthy food accessible and supplements visible (not hiding in a cupboard), keeping a diffuser with calming oils on my desk, and having a yoga mat and dumbbells ready to go. That way, those good-for-me behaviors are basically on autopilot.

At the end of the day, building up your motherhood toolbox is all about knowing yourself and what helps you recharge. It's not one-size-fits-all, so don't be afraid to get creative and customize it to your needs. We all have our own unique strengths, weaknesses, and challenges that we navigate on the daily. Whether it's journaling, meal prepping, or even just taking five minutes for a solo dance party, find what works for you and make it a priority.

One of my missions is to debunk the idea that being whole and well is a complicated and demanding process. *Trust* is paramount to believing our body can take care of itself. Medical paradigms that want us to rely on outside sources have stolen much of our agency. As Erin Holt, an integrative nutritionist, explains "the body always works in our favor... we just need to access our inner healer."[19] She talks about "self-sourcing" healing instead of out-sourcing to external authorities.

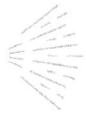 **WE CAN TAKE CARE OF OUR OWN WELLNESS WITH THE RIGHT BELIEFS, KNOWLEDGE, TOOLS, AND DAILY HABITS.**

I am going to share some knowledge and tools that I use with my clients. My purpose is to help you focus on priorities and give you some tangible action items to apply to your life. But remember, there is no right or wrong; choose what works for you. Also keep in mind how I taught you that stress is counterproductive; focus on gradual improvement and not perfection. Remember, what you are doing right now is easier because it is routine, so when you are making changes, it will take some initial extra effort. But with consistency and time that change will also become a habit. For additional information, including resources and virtual support, visit my website: www.carissastantonmd.com.

---

19 Liz Wolfe, host, "Be Your Own Health Expert and the Body-Belief Connection with The Funk'tional Nutritionist, Erin Holt," *Balanced Bites*, Episode 465, 5 August 2024. https://realfoodliz.com/balanced-bites-podcast-465-be-your-own-health-expert-and-the-body-belief-connection-with-the-funktional-nutritionist-erin-holt/

Pediatrician Tip: You can also use these tools to empower your children, not only by being an example, but also by encouraging them to take charge of their problems themselves. A child is having trouble falling asleep? Remind them to use deep breathing or a body scan meditation. A child is complaining of an itchy bug bite? Suggest they try an essential oil roller. Empowering children to help themselves not only relieves you of duties, but it improves their esteem. The goal is to teach children how to be independent beings—instead of handing them a fish, we should teach them *how* to fish.

sleep and stress management

I cannot say it enough—taking care of your nervous system is one of the most important things you can do for yourself. As I discussed in chapter 7, making sure you are not in constant survival mode is critical to physical and emotional well-being. Getting quality sleep and managing stress helps you maintain "rest-repair" mode. My dad is a mechanic, and of course he has to turn the engine off before he can fix it. Our bodies are the same—we need to downshift into rest to repair. Our bodies cannot fix themselves while running at high speed.

Improving sleep and managing stress had the most profound impact on my well-being, and I have seen it do the same with my clients. For me, it started with making sleep a priority. I implemented tools like cutting out blue light in the evenings, sticking to a consistent bedtime routine, and practicing relaxation techniques such as aromatherapy and meditation before bed. Slowly but surely, the quality of my sleep improved, which had a profound impact on my overall energy, mood, and ability to handle stress.

I also started experimenting with different methods to calm my nervous system during the day. By getting better at detecting when I was slipping into that survival mode and having strategies to counteract it (such as meditation and aromatherapy), I was able to spend more time in a parasympathetic "rest and repair" state. The results were remarkable. Rather than just existing in a state of exhaustion and reactivity, I began to feel genuinely resilient. My thyroid symptoms improved, my mental clarity sharpened, and I had more capacity to be truly present with my family. I wasn't just surviving; I was thriving.

I know what you're thinking. *How can I get sleep and manage stress when parenting is literally taking care of little ones around the clock?* It is ironic that two of the most important pillars of wellness are often the hardest to come by during this important season of life. But this comes back to what we taught you in parts I and II—you can find equilibrium between your needs and your family's needs. You can reduce the impact of motherhood on your nervous system by setting realistic boundaries and expectations, making space for yourself, and decluttering what does not serve you. And don't forget to take care of your physical health—the mind-body connection goes both ways; making the body healthy will also help the mind's regulation.

nutrition

When it comes to nutrition, there's no one-size-fits-all "right" way to eat healthy. It's more of a spectrum based on your personal values, resources, and family dynamics. The golden rule? Focus on getting as close to nature as possible. The more processed a food is, the less nutritious it tends to be and the more likely it is to have unhealthy additives. We also need to slow down and listen to our body by taking note of hunger cues, cravings, and how food makes us feel. I am keeping it simple here, but if you want more in-depth information, I recommend Liz Wolfe's insightful book *Eat the Yolks*.

Remember my attempt at healing my autoimmune disease with a strict diet that backfired? Keep in mind, the stress response diminishes your body's digestion process, which can make inflexible diets counterproductive. Here's the beauty of it: if you make your body resilient with healthy habits and regulate your nervous system, then you don't have to be perfect. Focus on making the majority of your diet as healthy as possible, and don't stress about the rest.

I know providing wholesome food for you and your family can be a large task. Remember to delegate and find shortcuts. For instance, I have my partner help with meal prep, such as cutting produce. During busy seasons I utilize a grocery delivery service that rescues food with imperfections and a meal delivery service that uses whole food ingredients. And if you have limited resources, then doing what you can to eat nutritiously is better than no effort at all. Remember that better is okay.

Even with a healthy diet, it can be difficult to get all the nutrients your body requires. High-quality supplements can also be a game-changer for filling in any nutritional gaps, so don't hesitate to work with a professional to find what works best for you. But keep it simple and prioritize; overthinking and overdoing can be counterproductive.

movement

Let's not forget the power of movement. A sedentary lifestyle doesn't just affect your physical health—it can take a toll on your mental and emotional well-being too. Aim to get your body moving for at least thirty minutes a day, whether that's a brisk walk, an impromptu dance party, or even some gentle stretching. And don't be afraid to get the kiddos involved too. They'll love the quality time and extra energy output.

Liz Wolfe, who is an expert in this area, would also encourage incorporating some strength and resistance training. Maintaining muscle mass is crucial for healthy aging and keeping your metabolism revved up. After all, muscles use more energy even when we are not using them. It does not need to be pumping iron in a gym—you can add ankle and wrist weights to your walking routine. Start small and find what works for you. Every little bit counts.

▷ **breathwork**

Here's an interesting one: did you know that optimal, healthy breathing is slow, deep, and through the nose? Yet in our modern, stressed-out world, many of us have developed dysfunctional breathing patterns. Think rapid, shallow breaths through the mouth, with our shoulders rising.

Not only is proper breathing technique important for physical well-being, but it can also have a profound impact on your mental and emotional state. So be mindful of how you're inhaling and exhaling, and don't hesitate to seek help from a professional like an oral myofunctional therapist if you're having trouble breathing through your nose.

▷ **mind/spirit**

As women, we often think that to be truly spiritual, we need to disconnect from our physical bodies. But the reality is quite the opposite—nurturing the mind-body connection is essential for holistic well-being.

Mind-Body Connection

Modern living's fast paced and high productivity lifestyle can come between our mind and our body, leaving our mind wandering and our body in a stress response. We need to intentionally reconnect our thoughts with our body, and vice versa. There are many ways to do this—deep breathing, yoga, and of course meditation.

One of the most powerful tools for aligning ourselves is meditation. Now, I know a lot of people have misconceptions about meditation, believing that it means to sit in silence and try to empty your mind. The first meditation class I attended was like this, but rather than being empty, my mind was focused on the snoring sound of someone who fell asleep during the class. But there are so many different styles and approaches, and it's important to find what feels best to you. At its core, meditation is the ability to focus attention and awareness to achieve a stable state with mental clarity and emotional calmness. Any activity that forces us to be present in the moment can be utilized, such as focusing on breathing, expressive writing, praying, or even doing a puzzle.

An easy place to start is a body scan meditation that focuses on awareness, sensations, and relaxing certain parts of the body, one at a time, typically from head to toe. This will help the mind tune into the body and integrate that mind-body awareness. One advantage of modern technology is the accessibility of virtual content such as videos of guided meditations, as well as other resources. I encourage you to explore and see what resonates. Even just a few minutes a day can make a world of difference.

Emotional Well-Being

Emotions are just that—energy in motion. If we feel an emotion, but we hide it or repress it, then that energy still exists. This is why crying when you are sad or exercising when you are angry helps you feel better—it helps that energy move. It is important to allow yourself to feel and process emotions, or else that energy can cause problems for your well-being.

We may have past emotional wounds that need to heal. Parenting is a continual self-improvement project because we are less able to hide our weaknesses—children are like mirrors reflecting our flaws. Addressing harmful imprints can be a heavy undertaking. We cannot cheat ourselves by going around them; we have to go through them to break down the false beliefs and rebuild new beliefs.

How do we go through those beliefs? Many times, it's necessary to revisit the initial trauma in our mind and process the repressed emotions. Trauma is not just about the events themselves but how our brains process and store those experiences. If we don't have adequate coping mechanisms in place, our minds can suppress those improve your well-being

emotions instead of allowing us to fully feel and work through them. There are specialized techniques designed to help us access the neurological pathways and stored energy and release those suppressed experiences in a safe, supported way. Many therapies are available such as energy work (Reiki), brainspotting, eye movement desensitization and reprocessing (EMDR), neuro-linguistic programming, and emotional freedom technique (EFT). There is not a right or wrong method; what works for the individual is a good choice. I've seen firsthand how transformative these modalities can be for deeper healing work.

Aromatherapy

In our modern, high-stress world, it's so easy for our brains to misinterpret everyday situations as threats, causing that fight-or-flight stress response. But there's a simple, natural tool that can help short-circuit this process: aromatherapy.

Certain plants, like lavender, make oils that have a grounding, calming effect on the amygdala, the part of the brain that senses danger. It's as if the scent tricks your body into thinking you're simply "stopping to smell the roses," rather than facing a real threat like running from a lion. Since your nose and nervous system are wired to recognize plant oil chemicals, aromatherapy with pure essential oils is more effective and safer than synthetic oils or fragrances. As a bonus, they can also be a useful natural tool to use with children, so you can take care of yourself and them as well.

Balance of Feminine and Masculine Energy

As women, we have this innate feminine energy—the receptive, intuitive, nurturing side of ourselves. But in our fast-paced, achievement-oriented culture, it can be easy to get stuck in a more masculine, outward-focused mode. This can not only interfere with our relationships, but also with our emotional well-being. For instance, the feminine side of us should be comfortable receiving, such as gifts or a massage from your partner. If accepting makes you uncomfortable, then the masculine energy is likely overriding the feminine.

Finding ways to consciously cultivate and honor that feminine essence is so vital for our mental, emotional, and spiritual health. Whether it's spending time in nature, receiving help from a partner, or engaging in more creative/expressive pursuits, these practices help us recharge those intuitive, receptive qualities.

At the same time, we also need to accept the masculine action-oriented, problem-solving side. We need to find that balance and flow between the two—the ying and the yang according to Chinese philosophy—so we can show up fully in all aspects of our lives.

environment

In our industrialized world, we're bombarded with toxins from all sides—in our food and water, personal care products, household cleaners, and the very air we breathe. And while it can feel overwhelming to try and eliminate every single source, taking a few strategic steps to reduce our overall toxic load can make a big difference.

The first and most important step is to focus on the basics that make our body more resilient: getting enough sleep, managing stress, and nourishing our bodies with whole, nutrient-dense foods. These foundational habits help strengthen our natural detoxification pathways.

From there, we can look at easy swaps for some of the most common culprits. For instance, trading out harsh chemical cleaners for gentler, plant-based alternatives can help our bodies and the environment. When it comes to personal care items like lotions, makeup, and soap, we can read labels and prioritize clean, non-toxic formulas.

While we can't control every single exposure, being mindful about the products we bring into our homes and bodies can go a long way.

improve your well-being

The most important thing to remember is that we don't have to be perfect. Small, sustainable changes are better than overwhelming ourselves with unrealistic standards. Every step we take to create a healthier environment is a win.

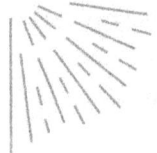

Take Home

CHAPTER 10
improve your well-being

◇ **Make yourself a priority.** Set boundaries and make yourself a priority to show yourself love and worthiness.
- When is the last time you did something just for yourself?
- If you are not able to do something for yourself daily, how can you start?
- What brings you joy, and how can you incorporate that into your life?

◇ **Find your equilibrium.** Balance is not always achievable, but we can maintain our function and wellness despite what is happening in our lives.
- Are you able to keep yourself functioning and well on a daily basis?
- If not, how can you improve your equilibrium?

◇ **Use wellness tools.** Develop a set of wellness modalities that help you maintain wellness.
- What tools do you currently use to help support your wellness?
- Are those working for you, or do you need new/more tools?
- What is one thing you can add to your wellness routine?

CHAPTER 11

makeover your motherhood
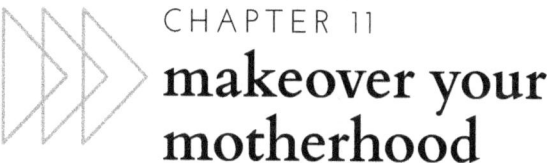

"There is no way to be a perfect mother, but a million ways to be a good one."

-Jill Churchill

small shifts make a big difference

Change isn't easy; I get it. It's simpler to stick with the status quo. But the status quo is not working for mothers or children.

To repeat a line from the introduction, many of us are stuck in a self-deprecating and overworking hamster wheel. We can find ourselves in a vicious loop where the very act of trying to be the "perfect" parent drains our capacity to regulate, undermines our emotional stability, and compromises our rational decision-making. Breaking this motherhood burnout cycle requires a multi-pronged approach. We can flip the arrows in a helpful direction at any point: decreasing our overwhelming commitments, increasing our self-care practices to increase our resilience, finding ways to short-circuit the triggered survival responses to improve logical thinking, and decreasing worry. But once we put a kink in the chain, the positive effects will unravel.

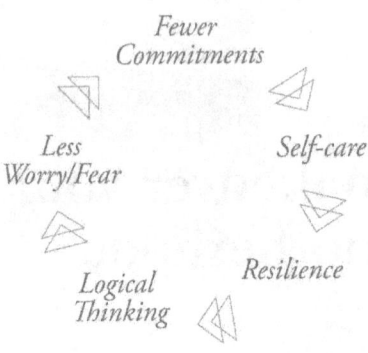

We have two options. One, we can continue this downward spiral of burnout, misalignment, and frustration, passing those ideals onto our children. Or two, we can declare that the buck stops here and break the cycle to realign our motherhood and our children's childhood.

WHEN SOMETHING ISN'T WORKING, WE HAVE THE CHOICE TO EITHER ACCEPT IT OR CHANGE IT.

Luckily, we are in the information era, where we have the knowledge and tools at our fingertips to transform our lives. You have the power to change your experience and journey.

Reconciling where we are with where we want to be may seem insurmountable. But remember that small shifts can make a big difference. What you're doing now is easy because it's routine, and initial change takes extra effort. But you can do hard things. You can persevere until the change becomes routine. And don't try to change too much at once—focus on one goal, and when that becomes routine, move to the next. Be patient with the process.

I always remind myself, "Rome wasn't built in a day." Your changes don't have to be huge. You do not necessarily need to uproot your life all at once. We can find ways to reclaim parts we've lost in modern living while still living in modern times.

I recently attended a retreat with a group of mothers. We were in a circle dancing with a local instructor leading us. One mother was holding her nine-month-old infant, and when the mothers started dancing, the baby began kicking her legs and clapping her hands. This spontaneous communion was reminiscent of the scene in the documentary *Babies* where the African child joins a group of mothers in tribal dancing. You don't have to move to another country to reclaim motherhood; you can find your own way right here, right now.

you've got this!

I hope this book validates your problems, shifts your perception, and empowers you to redefine your own motherhood and resist forces working against that definition. If we each take steps to improve the narrative, we can raise the collective of mothers for generations to come.

As you reach the end of the journey we've been on together throughout this book, it's time to put what you've learned into practice. This is your opportunity to truly take charge of your motherhood experience and create the life you desire.

First and foremost, take a hard look at your current reality and make some critical evaluations. What aspects of your life are no longer serving you? What beliefs, habits, or commitments are weighing you down? It's time to courageously let go of anything that is holding you back.

As a pediatrician, one of the most important things I do is give mothers permission to take steps in this process. So though you don't *need* my permission, here it is: it is okay to let go of something that does not serve you and your family. If the benefit of an activity or obligation doesn't outweigh the risk to your family's overall health and happiness, then it's time to make a different choice. Remember, if something is causing unnecessary stress and negatively affecting your well-being, then it is likely counterproductive to the goal of connection with your child. This is why self-sacrifice is a false narrative. Absolve yourself of the fear of "scarring a child for life" if you go against the social norm. I promise you, the lasting impact of a thriving, fulfilled mother will be far more profound.

The path of motherhood is never a predictable straight line. There will be ups and downs, times when you need to be more vigilant and attentive, and others when you can afford to step back. And of course, if you're going through a personal difficulty or transition, don't hesitate to call in the reinforcements of your village and utilize any shortcuts or hacks that can lighten your load. As a working mom, my own family knows I'm fighting to keep my equilibrium when the crockpot meals and paper plates come out. Remember that no motherhood journey is perfect, but it unfolds perfectly how it was meant to. Give yourself grace and credit that you are doing the best you can, which is all your child needs.

> I will tell you, my journey was not flawless. It started in the throes of demanding medical school training. There were several years of single parenting in the middle, followed by a blended family transition. Throughout I fell into some of the narratives and "traps" we talked about in this book. I blindly followed unreasonable expectations, self-sacrifice, and perfectionism, which led to minimal time for myself and caused my well-being to suffer. Ultimately, my motherhood makeover was not what I did for my daughter; it was what I did for myself. I sought continual growth and improvement. I do have repressed emotional trauma (events my body was not

allowed or able to process at the time), so unveiling that and a softening of myself needed to happen. But at the same time, I regained my own power and confidence. None of this happened overnight or easily. It was a gradual and intentional process. My breakthrough came when I started to set boundaries, let go of expectations, and make space for myself. Then I realized how good it felt to be parenting from a calm mode instead of a reactionary one. And in the end, I am a better person because of my daughter, and she is who she was meant to be. So although the journey is imperfect, the destination is what counts.

Keep this mantra in mind: Everything is "figure-out-able." Trust that whatever comes next, you have the power to navigate anything. Have faith, when you are in the thick of parenting's challenges, that nothing lasts forever; this too shall pass. Ultimately, remember that even after doing (and not doing) all the things, so much of life is outside of our control. I've seen it time and time again as a doctor—even when parents do everything "perfectly," their child may not have the desired outcomes. And conversely, I've witnessed children who have had an abusive or neglectful childhood, and yet they manage to grow into resilient, thriving adults. It's both humbling and frustrating, isn't it? Life, and motherhood, is more about letting things unfold than forcing them to happen.

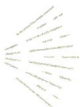
RADICAL ACCEPTANCE IS A BELIEF THAT CAN SHIFT OUR FOCUS FROM WHAT WE DO NOT CONTROL TO WHAT WE CAN CONTROL.

This point of view can have a profound effect on our perception and experience. Instead of being motivated by fear (remember FOMO parenting), we can be a secure and sure parent with a sense of ease and peace.

What do we control then? Our actions and reactions—and you can start now. Go back to the end of each chapter to review the key points and action items. Make a list of your goals, the barriers to those goals, and the little shifts you can make one at a time. Those incremental changes will add up to a monumental difference in your motherhood experience.

The path forward is yours to decide—you have the power to steer your own journey through the barriers and towards sustainability, peace, and fulfillment. It is time to makeover *your* motherhood. You've got this!

Take Home

CHAPTER 11
makeover your motherhood

◇ **Make small shifts.** You can take steps to reconcile where you are and where you want to be.
- What is one area where you can flip the arrow on the cycle of motherhood burnout: decreasing commitments, increasing self-care practices, finding ways to short-circuit the triggered survival responses, or decreasing your fear and worry?
- What is one action item you can do today to improve that area?

◇ **Makeover your motherhood.** You have the power to make your life what you want it to be.
- What is an area that is not serving you or your family?
- How can you let go or modify this area?
- What are the barriers to that change and how can you break through?

acknowledgements

This book would not have been possible without my village. I am honored to have you in my life and cannot thank you enough.

I am grateful for my family and friends:
    Kathryn Garey-my extraordinary daughter and greatest inspiration
    Jerod Stanton-my soul mate and greatest support
    Allison Stanton-my bonus daughter and kind heart
    Reese Stanton-my bonus daughter and positive spirit
    Pam Langenfeld-my mother and courageous cycle-breaker
    Ken Langenfeld-my father and dependable rock
    Rebecca Dyro-my mama bear friend and lifeline
    Beth Switzenberg-my lifelong friend and confidant

I am grateful for my colleagues:
    Liz Wolfe for her insight and direction
    Tara Haddon for her intuitive healing
    Jessica Yeager for her transformative sharing
    Danielle Yeager for her inspiration
    Cody Skinner for her empathy
    Liz Levy for her solidarity
    Kendra Rose for her caring
    Jennifer Osgood for her wisdom
    Victoria Weber for her nourishment
    Stephanie Risinger for her expertise
    Kerri Nachlas for her fairy godmother skills
    Erin Boje for her vision
    Erin Wisemore for her teamwork

I am grateful for the team at Streamline Books:
　Will and Lauren Severns for their ingenuity
　Chloie Benton for her writing talent
　Abigael Elliott for her artistic talent
　Cindy Venable for her editing expertise
　Alice Briggs for her design skills

I am grateful for those who shared their journey:
　Shawn Manenye
　Phil and Manju Abraham
　Carolyn Young
　Christine White
　Faith North
　Whitney Webb
　Megan Hettich

www.ingramcontent.com/pod-product-compliance
Lightning Source LLC
Chambersburg PA
CBHW020546030426
42337CB00013B/990